CONQUERING
PAIN

The Art of Healing
with BioMagnetism

Award Winning Therapy Book
Advanced Healing & Well Being

Peter Kulish

CONQUERING PAIN: The Art of Healing with BioMagnetism

Copyright © 1999, 2016 by Peter Kulish

First Edition published April 1999, Reprint 2003, 2008, Second Edition published 2016

The information contained in this book describes various Biomagnetic energy techniques and protocols that are based on successful clinical therapies that have been used worldwide for many years.

In the quest to provide a better quality of life for humanity, Peter Kulish in conjunction with the Foundation for Magnetic Science and its BiomagScience® Research has compiled the following Biomagnetic information and protocols for those individuals who wish to learn more about the complementary use of magnetic energy medicine for health and healing.

This information is provided as an educational tool for complementary health therapies. It is intended as an educational adjunct to a physician and/or caregiver's advice or treatment.

Individuals with health problems should consult with their health-care providers before administering any therapies suggested in this book. Any application of the materials set forth in the following pages is done at the reader's discretion and is his or her sole responsibility. Your health and well-being are important to us. We trust you will benefit from this information on biomagnetism.

ISBN: 978-0-692-69254-7

Email: Office@biomagscience.net
www.BiomagScience.net
215-862-6777

Published by
Fountainville Press
Fountainville, Pennsylvania

CONTENTS

This book is dedicated to:
The great healing energy medicine of Biomagnetism
And all people who strive to use it for a better quality life.

Active in Research and Development since 1979, under the auspices of the Foundation for Magnetic Science, BiomagScience (formerly Magnetizer Biomagnetic Laboratories) has led in the evolution of Biomagnetism to create the most powerful, lightweight, certified BioMagnets and the most advanced, step-by-step scientific therapy protocols to address over 170 simple, acute and chronic medical conditions. Our research and associated practitioners, clinics, and medical institutions are devoted to providing the extraordinary science of Biomagnetic Energy Medicine and its ability to support and rapidly progress the body's healing mechanisms.

Through years of research, therapeutic development, and worldwide application of BiomagScience energy techniques, BiomagScience's protocols have demonstrated remarkable results on most medical conditions including breakthroughs that read like miracles. Besides helping quickly resolve conditions like carpal tunnel syndrome, arthritis or chronic back pain, some protocols have awoken people from terminating comas, helped heal crushed splintered bones in two and half months instead of ten, regenerated severed nerves, helped resolve mid-stage MS, rebuilt herniated discs to full height; and the list goes on. These results are occurring every day throughout the world and are based on utilizing the correct magnetic field application to jump start and amplify the body's own natural healing.

The objective of this book is to provide the reader with the fundamentals and the most advanced Biomagnetic energy techniques available to help and enhance the body's ability to resolve pain, overcome illness and injury, increase wellness and vitality, and preserve optimal health.

Best of Health!
Peter Kulish

Acknowledgments

It is with great thanks to some very special people who spent their lives researching, developing and teaching the various energy medicine disciplines and the scientific precepts of Biomagnetism that made it possible to create this significant therapy book about the precise basic and advanced protocols of how to help resolve over 170 simple, acute, chronic and complex medical conditions.

To Cathy Moore, Co-Editor and former Director of Biomagnetic Laboratories (now BiomagScience) for her knowledge of publishing, nutrition, and physiology in helping create this book.

To Phillip Schaeffer, Senior Advisor and Co-Editor, former Director of the Royal Society of Medicine, and lecturer for the United Nations International Trade Commission, whose sage-like presence gave us the clarity and focus to bring this project to completion.

To Tom Levy, M.D., Nutritional researcher extraordinaire, for the wonderful truth about nutrition and health.

To Karen McChrystal, MA, Editor, Second Edition, for her guidance and great help.

To the wonderful family of friends, researchers, and practitioners worldwide, who continue to contribute to this remarkable and admirable science.

And to my family, who is my fortune.

For any further information on white papers, before and after cellular research, case studies, additional health conditions, FAQs, and a myriad of additional information, go to www.BiomagScience.net.

QUICK REFERENCE GUIDE

Proper Polarity Placement For Pain Therapy

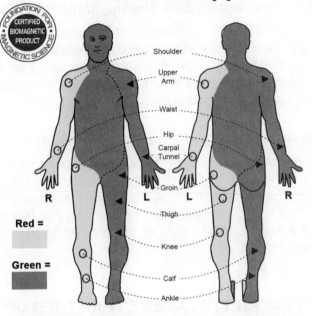

Green = Negative Meridian Red = Positive Meridian
Do Not Use BioMagnets In Red Zone.. Always in Green Zone
except for Advanced Circuit Therapy

What is Pain?

Pain is the response to damage and disorganization of cellular functions and nerve connections occurring from inflammation from stress or trauma.

How Does Biomagnetism Help Pain?

BioMagnetism substantially amplifies the body's normal healing energy which reduces inflammation immediately while reorganizing the distressed metabolism and nerve functions, resulting in reducing and eliminating pain.

Why Is Negative (Green) Side Therapy Used for Pain?

Science has found that when a stressed or traumatized site goes into a healing mode, the site naturally becomes electro-negatively charged. The BioMagnet's green colored Bio-Negative field immediately amplifies the site's natural healing energy to rapidly eliminate pain and increase healing.

What Are the Energy Meridians of the Body?

Science has identified the body's normal energy patterns in the limbs and throughout the body. In the above anatomical (thumbs out) illustration, the right side front (anterior) and the left side back (posterior) of the limbs, shoulders and hips are all Positive (red) meridians. The exact opposite side of these body locations are Negative (green) meridians.

PROPER POLARITY PLACEMENT for THERAPY

Why Are Meridians Important in Therapy?

The meridians of the limbs and shoulders are like the battery in your car or electronic device. The polarity can never be reversed because it will spark and short circuit. The same is true when applying a BioMagnet on the limbs of the human body. The BioMagnet's Bio-Negative (green) healing side must be placed using the Proper Polarity Placement on the Negative (green) meridian to amplify the body's proper energy flow for quick relief. With a slight exception [noted below], applying the Bio-Negative (green) energy on the Positive (red) meridian will cause stress and often starts to hurt after 30 minutes.

Pain Therapy in the Positive Red Meridian

When the pain occurs in the Positive (red) meridian, simply place the BioMagnet's Bio-Negative (green) side exactly on the opposite side of the limb on the Negative (green) meridian on the shoulders, hands, feet, wrists, ankles, etc. This will properly amplify the body's natural Negative healing energy into the Positive (red) meridian and provide rapid pain relief.

Two exceptions to applying the Bio-Negative green on a Positive red meridian: 1. A single Power Wafer may be used for a cut, scrape, burn or bakers cyst for 20 Minutes ONLY, then must be removed. 2. May be used on the hip anywhere, except when Circuit Therapy is applied.

NOTE: Most people feel pain after applying the Bio-Negative (green) side on the Positive (red) meridian for 30 minutes; it stresses and prohibits healing.

If the PAIN is in the Negative (green) meridian, directly apply the Bio-Negative (green) side directly on the site.

If the PAIN is in the Positive (red) meridian, apply the Bio-Negative (green) on the opposite side of the pain in the green meridian for proper therapy, pain relief and rapid healing.

Examples:

- Carpal Tunnel pain on the right wrist requires Bio-Negative (green) on the top of the wrist (posterior, opposite palm side) opposite the pain.
- If the pain is in the Positive meridian of the right front (anterior) ankle, knee, elbow or shoulder, etc., apply the Bio-Negative (green) side on the back (posterior) side just opposite the pain.
- If the pain is in the Positive meridian of the left back (posterior) ankle, knee, elbow or shoulder, etc., apply the Bio-Negative (green) side on the front (anterior) just opposite the pain.

- If the pain is on the side of a Positive meridian front (anterior), apply the Bio-Negative on the opposite side on the Negative meridian.

BiomagScience requires proper placement to correctly amplify the body's natural energies. This is necessary to ensure the increase in cellular vitality levels necessary to provide rapid pain relief and healing.

World Leader in BiomagScience

www.BiomagScience.Net

STORY OF THE HEART
BY PETER KULISH

"You may know someone who is suffering from an illness.
This is about someone very special to me, who was suffering."

Dear Readers,

Many years ago, I became very interested in how magnetism could help the body heal. This led me to the great researcher Dr. Albert Roy Davis, the godfather of contemporary biomagnetics. Many years ago Dr. Davis had discovered the basic, scientific, biomagnetic precepts that researchers further developed and are using today. It was my honor to have known and studied with him.

In 1979, I began my own research into the field of Biomagnetism and Magnetic Physics. As a result, BiomagScience under the Foundation for Magnetic Science (formerly Magnetizer Scientific Research Institute) was formed. The Biomagnetic focus of the foundation was to scientifically understand the physiological electrical nature of cells and tissue and how magnetic fields could help amplify the cells and the body back to health. Within a short period of time, we realized how significant our findings could be for people everywhere.

Through the years, BiomagScience research has led in the development of advanced magnetic therapies and protocols that have helped people with such conditions as lupus, carpal tunnel syndrome, CFS, MS, and most other acute and chronic illness and disease. It's a wonderful feeling to see someone who is extremely ill apply a sequence of small, powerful magnets and return to health. When used properly, biomagnetism has been shown to be one of the greatest complimentary therapeutic breakthroughs of all time.

Perhaps destiny played a role when disaster hit home in my family. The doctors of Dupont Children's Hospital diagnosed someone very dear to me, an 11-month-old little baby girl, with an aggressive case of hemihypertrophy – Elephant Man's Disease. This is a rare disease where one hemisphere (one half of the body, from head to toe) uncontrollably outgrows the other half of the body.

I asked the doctors what could be done and they told me that periodically, as she grew unevenly, they could cut out sections of bone from her arm and leg to shorten them. During the bone re-sectioning, they also would cut out sections of her flesh, which they said would give her a "somewhat normal life."

Totally taken aback, I couldn't believe what I was hearing. I asked them what caused it. They had no idea, but considered it a genetic disorder. I went home and was terribly upset as I thought about the child having to suffer through all these procedures.

Upon further research about Elephant Man's Disease and after seeing detailed photos of adults with deformities, I understood why modern medicine would resection the body. Otherwise, it was too unimaginable to think about.

Further research explained how the DNA's genetic code was transmitted between the transmitter and receptor sites and how the growth hormone coding is signaled from the brain through the nervous system into the cells and much more.

While reading volumes of medical research I came across shingles – painful blisters caused by the active varicella virus known as chicken pox which can lie dormant for years, but can reactivate when the immune system is low, causing an outbreak of shingles to show up on one side (hemisphere) of the body. This would indicate the virus finds a home on one side the body, and since the central nervous system is what transmits the growth hormone communication, I assumed the virus must attach itself to one side of the spine.

After seven months of research, I felt I was getting somewhere. I recalled that the child's mother had contracted chicken pox in her fifth month of pregnancy! Apparently, a high population of this virus was residing on the child's spine and acting as a genetic junk filter that was not allowing the growth hormone signal to properly transmit evenly to both sides of the baby's body.

By the time I learned this, the little girl was 18 months old and the large bone structure of her left hemisphere was approximately 17% larger than her right, as accurately measured by bone-growth x-ray tests. The frightening issue was that the left side of her forehead was starting to bulge and her left hand and foot were almost twice the size of her right hand and foot.

Having studied and worked with the viral and bacterial responses to increased blood oxygen and Vitamin C, I immediately started oxygen and Vitamin C therapy (mentioned later in this book) to help kill the viral population. I also ran nutritional lab tests to see what nutrients she might need for complete nutrition.

Finally, I applied the most important therapy: two small, Rare Earth Powered BioMagnets, facing Bio-Negative to the skin, on the spine on the lower back of her neck. I had studied, developed, and had applied similar therapies for post-stroke, MS, neurosis, depression, and ankylosing spondylitis. Now I applied the Bio-Negative magnetic field to lyse (kill) the virus. I felt this magnetic therapy might reduce or eliminate the viral population causing the condition and that the electromotive energy might also help her to be able to equalize the left and right-brain hemispheres, which might start rebalancing the growth issues to help normalize the little girl.

By the age of 6, her right side growth had caught up and she had become fully balanced. Today, she is a healthy, attractive adult.

Now you know how important Biomagnetism has been to my family and the kind of science and foundational background that have helped in developing the therapies and protocols that has helped so many throughout the world. I have compiled this book so that you can learn how the complimentary therapies of Biomagnetism may help you and your family to increase their vitality, overcome pain and illness, and achieve wellness from most injuries and medical conditions.

Peter Kulish

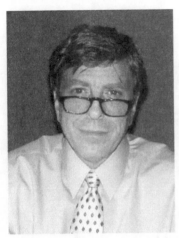

Peter Kulish began his research in bio-magnetic therapy over three decades ago. Originally studying and consulting with the godfather of biomagnetism, Albert Roy Davis, Peter took an advanced degree from the Broeringmeyer BioMagnetic Institute and has consulted, and developed energy medicine protocols with doctors, scientists, and researchers from around the globe.

He is respected worldwide for his extensive research of Biomagnetism and pioneering the development of advanced therapies and protocols for prevention, wellness and resolution of pain, injury, illness, disease, nerve regeneration and most medical conditions.

Extensively researched and used by the Asian Energy Medicine Association, his protocols are taught in curricula throughout Asia, where Energy Medicine is considered standard medical practice. His therapies are also used by individuals, practitioners, and in medical institutions and health spas throughout the world.

As a master healer with a wealth of over thirty years of research and application in the effects of magnetism on all aspects of the human body, he has been a featured guest speaker on biomagnetism at clinics, hospitals, medical colleges, and universities and has been interviewed extensively on TV and radio, headlining many times on the "International Science Hour."

This new, more comprehensive second edition of Conquering Pain includes additional information, before and after research findings, and case studies. It explains further how Biomagnetism works and provides new, advanced Biomagnetic therapy protocols, not in the former edition, that have successfully helped overcome medical conditions.

5

CHAPTER ONE

MAGNETIC FIELD THERAPY

The use of magnets to generate controlled electromotive stimulating fields has many medical applications and has proven to be one of the most effective means for diagnosing and helping resolve pain, illness and disease. Used widely in other parts of the world, it is just now starting to be recognized by Western medicine as a valuable therapy in treating physical and emotional disorders.

According to Wolfgang Ludwig, Sc.D., Ph.D., Director of the Institute for Biophysics in Horb, Germany, "Magnetic field therapy is a method that penetrates the whole human body and can treat every organ without chemical side effects." Magnetic field therapy has been used effectively for the following conditions:

- Rheumatoid disease
- Infections and inflammation
- Headaches and migraines
- Insomnia and sleep disorders
- Circulatory problems
- Fractures and pain
- Environmental stress
- Nerve and tissue regeneration

How Magnetic Field Therapy Works

"The healing potential of magnets is possible because the body's nervous system is governed, in part, by varying patterns of ionic currents and electromagnetic fields," reports Dr. Zimmerman, Ph.D. (former President of the Bio-Electric-Magnetics Institute).

BiomagScience has determined that proper magnetic fields are able to penetrate the body and affect the functioning of the cells of the glands, organs, hard and soft tissue, and the nervous system by aggressively increasing their cellular electrical voltage (electromotive vitality), resulting in electromotively forcing the cells to increase their metabolic and immune functions. The increased cellular energy results in helping the body quickly reduce pain and resolve most health conditions while achieving and maintaining wellness.

When used properly, magnetic field therapy has no harmful side effects. This book is about how to use Biomagnetism correctly.

All Magnets Have Two Poles

One is South, and the other North. As there are conflicting methods of naming the poles of a magnet, such as the seeking pole, a magnetometer and a gaussmeter are used as a standard method to determine which side is emitting Positive (Geo South) or Negative (Geo North) electromotive energies. If a compass is used to locate the poles of the magnet, the needle pointing to the "Geological North Pole" of the earth will also point to the magnet's Negative (Geo North) pole, and vice versa.

Research worldwide teaches that the Bio-Negative energy amplifies the body's own natural healing energy which naturally reduces inflammation and increases cellular metabolic and immune functions producing a calming, healing, alkalizing and normalizing effect. In contrast, the Bio-Positive pole has a stressful, inflammatory effect and with prolonged exposure, produces acidity, reduces cellular oxygen, supports anaerobic bacteria and reduces normal metabolic functioning. The Bio-Positive energy is used carefully and generally in conjunction with the Bio-Negative energy in advanced therapies.

How Magnets Are Used Therapeutically

Magnetic therapy can be applied in many ways. Devices range from small, solid-state magnets to large machines capable of generating high magnitudes of field strength (used for treating fractures and conditions like MS). In various parts of the world, magnetic devices are medically recognized, quite popular and covered by medical insurance. BiomagScience's research has determined that solid state magnets offer the only magnetic energy applications that work in the same sympathetic energy level as the body's cells. Subsequently BiomagScience has developed the most extensive and comprehensive advances in supportive healing by synergistically amplifying the cell's own healing energy for the required condition.

BiomagScience BioMagnets can be placed individually or on multiple locations on the body, in the privacy of your home, and this book provides all the techniques and protocols that have helped people throughout the world achieve rapid pain relief and heal over 170 simple, acute and chronic conditions.

Conditions Benefited by Magnetic Field Therapy

Therapies can last from just a few minutes to a few months, and depending upon the severity of the condition, may be applied throughout the day and/or night. Most health conditions can be addressed with magnetic therapy and sometimes with miracle-like results on acute injury, chronic illness or disease: BiomagScience cites cases of people awakening from terminating comas, regeneration of severed nerves or crushed bones healing four hundred percent faster.

In a case cited by Dr. Wolfgang Ludwig, a forty-six-year-old man, had suffered for years from severe heart flutter, diarrhea, and nausea. Nothing helped until a low-gauss magnet was placed upon his solar plexus for only three minutes; his symptoms immediately ceased. After two years, he still had experienced no relapse.

In another case described by Dr. William Philpott, a seventy-year-old man, continued to suffer from heart pain after undergoing coronary bypass surgery. His speech slurred, he walked with a shuffle, and lived in a state of chronic depression. He decided to try magnetic therapy, and a biomagnet was placed over his heart. Within ten minutes the pain disappeared. Magnets were then also applied to the crown of his head while he slept, and within a month, his depression was gone, his speech was clear, and his walking returned to normal.

BiomagScience confirms the findings that Biomagnetism helps eliminate toothaches, periodontal disease, and eradicate fungal infections like candidiasis; helps dissolve kidney stones and calcium deposits in inflamed tissue, and is particularly effective in reducing inflammation and edema. According to Dr. Philpott, "Symptoms of cardiac and brain atherosclerosis have been observed to disappear after six to eight weeks of nightly exposure to a Negative solid-state magnetic field." BiomagScience's case of arterial stenosis (calcium buildup in the heart) was eliminated in 6 weeks.

BiomagScience has shown that elevating the cellular voltage of an individual causes an immediate increase in health and vitality. Citing two cases of middle-aged women who were very ill with malabsorption, a condition in which the cells become stuck with such low energy (voltage), they were unable to absorb enough nutrition, oxygen and electrolytes to increase their cellular voltage to be able to become well.

Typical of malabsorption, they both suffered from chronic fatigue syndrome, fibromyalgia, and candidiasis and were bedridden for 15 and 25 years. Nothing allopathic or alternative, including poorly designed magnets, helped, and any nutritional supplement created a toxic reaction because the cells did not have the energy to metabolize the nutrition which the body then treated as a toxin. Using the BiomagScience lower CVS application (back of the neck at the hairline), both individuals immediately started healing within an hour of application. Using additional magnetic therapy, both individuals fully recovered; the woman who had been bedridden for 25 years was able to play competitive tennis within a year of the therapy (see cases under Research at www.BiomagScience.Net.)

Another case with outstanding results following BiomagScience proper placement on the body's meridians (See "Polarity Placement," pg. 138) is the 72-year-old man who, in a head-on collision, crushed both knees and splintered both legs down to his ankles, just before Thanksgiving. After the surgery, the doctors told him he would have to heal until August before he could start physiotherapy to learn to walk again. As a colleague knowledgeable about BiomagScience protocols, he immediately put Super BioMagnets down the front of his left leg and the back of his right. As a result, he did not need any pain medicine and was walking normally by the third week of January, having healed four times faster and without pain medications as the Biomagnets eliminated the pain.

The OGE (organ group energizing) therapy was created due to an unusual case. A fellow contacted us to find out if anything could be done for his 91-year-old father; his kidneys had failed so badly, dialysis could no longer be performed and he slipped into a septic shock coma.

Realizing that his primary organs were failing, we advised placing our Regular Size [Rare Earth Super] BioMagnets on the pancreas/spleen, right side of the liver and both kidneys, and a 2-Stack of Power Wafers on the lower CVS (the back of the neck at the hairline) to energize the brain. The supposition was that if we could energetically elevate all his primary organs at the same time, they might normalize in unison and bring his father back from the brink of death.

Three days later, instead of terminating as the trend indicated, his father woke up, his kidneys started to heal and he no longer needed dialysis. The fellow continued to live for a reasonable period of time, and when he died, it was naturally in his sleep. From this case, the OGE therapy was born and is now commonly used for other acute and chronic issues.

These are just a few of the many outstanding results that have resulted from the development and proper use of Biomagnetism. For more results, please see our BioMagnificent testimonials and cases in this book or our voluminous results at www.BiomagScience.Net web site.

Stress

BiomagScience concurs with Dr. Philpott that the Bio-Negative energy applied to the top of the head stimulates the pineal gland to naturally increase the hormone melatonin, which has a calming and sleep-inducing effect on brain and body functions. Melatonin has not only been shown to be anti-stressful, anti-aging, anti-infectious, anti-cancerous, and the first catalyst in restoration of the body, but it also helps heal free-radical sites (see before and after free-radical site healing Research at www.BiomagScience.Net).

Free radicals are Positively charged, highly destructive, oxidative molecules that, missing an electron, bond and destroy healthy tissue to balance the missing electron.* An excess of free radicals creates a decreased efficiency of protein synthesis and metabolic functions, which leads to premature aging of the cells, wrinkling of skin, hardening of the vascular system, illness and many other poor health conditions.

Since Bio-Negative energy neutralizes the positive energy of free radicals, it helps heal the multitude of conditions related to oxidative stress, infections, and aging from an excess of free radicals. For that reason, Biomagnetic therapy should be considered an important daily energy supplement for maintaining good health by eliminating this naturally occurring problem.

Bacterial, Fungal, and Viral Infections

"A Negative magnetic field can function like an antibiotic in helping destroy bacterial, fungal, and viral infections," says Dr. Philpott, "by promoting oxygenation and lowering the body's acidity." Both of these factors are beneficial to normal cellular functions but harmful to pathogenic (disease-causing) micro-organisms which do not survive in a well-oxygenated, alkaline environment. It has been proven that the biological value of oxygen is increased by the influence of a Negative magnetic field and that increasing the charge in a low energy cell will cause its Negative charged DNA (deoxyribonucleic acid) to "pull" more oxygen out of the bloodstream and into the cell. The Negative magnetic field helps promote and maintain the cellular buffer system (pH acid-base balance) and support healthy cellular alkalinity. The low-acid alkaline balance helps maintain the presence of oxygen in the body.

Author's note: The body naturally produces free radicals and receives many more free radicals in the form of toxins in the air, water, and food. The normal Positive electron spin of the oxidative free radical that damages healthy tissue is systemically and rapidly neutralized and healed with the proper Bio-Negative energy of a BioMagnet. See "free radicals" in the research appendix.

The Future of Magnetic Field Therapy

BiomagScience worldwide research and case studies confirm Dr. Philpott's report that the application of Bio-Negative magnetic fields provide the most predictable results of any therapy he has observed. "It is not only valuable as a medically supervised technique, but works well for many self-help problems such as insomnia, chronic pain, and tension."

Additionally because magnets do not introduce any foreign substance into the body, this makes them safer than long-term medications, and after 36 years of research and development of advanced therapies, BiomagScience energy medicine is a simple to use, scientifically based therapy that provides major pain relief and healing of conditions heretofore not able to be successfully addressed with allopathic medicine.

Author's note: Dr. Philpott has, like many reputable biomagnetic research-ers, subscribed to Albert R. Davis' initial precepts on single pole cellular responses. He is widely recognized for his biomagnetic research and devel-opment in such areas as cancer, diabetes and psychosis.

This part of the chapter is reprinted with permission from Burton Gold-berg: Alternative Medicine, the Definitive Guide ISBN# 0-9636334-3-0 www. alternativemedicine.com.

CHAPTER TWO

BRIEF HISTORY

Biomagnetics is not some kind of quasi- or pseudo-science. It is a science with a background of over 5,000 years' worth of research and use. The employment of magnetism in healing has been traced back to 3000 B.C. in documented Chinese medicine using lodestones (natural occurring magnets) for healing.

In Ancient Egypt, medical practitioners used the lodestones. At the time considered to be supernatural, their form of medicine by today's standards would most likely be called holistic. Although denied credit for their contributions, Pharonic medicine influenced many ancient civilizations, such as the Greek and Roman. Cleopatra used a magnetic lodestone for sleeping on and indicated she attributes her beauty to it.

Malta, another one of the ancient Eastern cultures, also embraced this necessary art of healing from Egypt. The Maltese Order is considered to be the successor of the Egyptian Priesthood and the emissaries of this ancient wisdom. Their secrets in healing were preserved and passed on from parent to child, down the lineage, to one noteworthy individual who was advancing an unorthodox form of medicine, relating new scientific definitions to the ancient occult knowledge.

Paracelsus, born in 1493, also known as the Father of Medicine, was a direct descendant of the Grand Prior of the Knights of Malta. Thus, he was instructed by his father in the secrets of this ancient medicine and combined the mysteries of Egyptian healing with modern education. Around the year 1515 he obtained his Doctorate at the University of Ferrara and prepared himself against attacks that he knew would be coming from peers within the orthodox medical field.

He is the first scientist known to make clear the distinction between medicine and chemistry, thereby removing the aura of mystery surrounding alchemy and providing further explanation of his use of magnetics for healing. He went on to publish innumerable articles on healing with herbs and magnets, providing the public with prescriptions and instructions for diagnosis.

In his book, he described the causes and origins of disease and in other published articles, detailed explanation of the forces radiated by magnets. His aim was to treat the actual cause of the disease and heal it with magnets, thereby alleviating the symptoms at the same time, practicing what we now call Biomagnetism. Indeed, he was among the first to describe how the chemical balance within the internal environment of the human body was directly influenced by magnetism.

The most unusual, if not the most spectacular use of magnets is described by Paracelsus in connection with therapy for epilepsy, or as he terms it, "the falling disease in which you stand up and everything rushes to the top of your head." According to his method, the patient is laid on his stomach and the disease, which is centered in the top of the head, is driven by means of the magnets to the solar plexus. We have since used magnetic therapy on the neck/brain which has helped stop epileptic seizures. (See testimonials, Chapter 13.)

Paracelsus continually recommended magnetic therapy for relieving pains such as cramps and spasms caused by tetanus or in childbirth. He also used magnets extensively for therapy for jaundice, piles and hernia, stating in regards to hernia, "the magnet draws the rupture together in a most wonderful way and is effective with both young and old."

Unfortunately, Paracelsus' peers viewed his publications as unorthodox – hardly surprising since he mercilessly criticized the medical profession of his day. The campaign that he waged against orthodox colleagues escalated to a pitched battle in which he was only able to save his life by taking flight.

Through a combination of science and the ancient Egyptian mysteries, Paracelsus was able to gain insight and knowledge to treat the causes of diseases. Although ahead of his time, Paracelsus pioneered a new form of holistic medicine that was based on chemistry. Like the Chinese, he treated the cause, not the symptoms, his methods effecting a cure. In 1541 Paracelsus died at the hands of those who thought him a madman.

Fortunately science has made significant strides in understanding the fundamentals of cellular energy and how an external magnetic field can affect cellular health.

In the 1930s, scientist Albert Roy Davis distinguished the different effects that the North (Bio-Negative) and South (Bio-Positive) fields of a magnet have upon the biological systems of humans and animals. He developed thousands of experiments which have led to the fundamental scientific precepts that have been used to establish the correct biomagnetic protocols (therapy) for humans and animals.

Finding that magnets had an effect on arthritis, glaucoma, aging, tumors and many other diseases, Davis concluded that the Bio-Negative magnetic field has an arresting, calming, and healing effect, while the Positive field has an aggressive and often stressful metabolic effect.

These precepts have led researchers to creating a large body of evidence of how cellular physiology is affected by energy therapy. Coupled with that information and the advances in technology, before and after cellular energy measurement, clinical studies, and a host of associate researchers worldwide, BiomagScience, under the guidance of Peter Kulish, has been able to develop some of the most advanced energy medicine therapies for supportive healing of conditions heretofore never achieved.

BiomagScience is recognized as a leader in advanced biomagnetic therapies. Its protocols are used by individuals and practitioners worldwide and are taught in curricula in Asian medical colleges, universities, and clinics where magnetic energy therapy is considered normal medicine.

CHAPTER THREE

Introduction to BioMagnetics

Although Biomagnetism dates back 5000 years throughout many cultures, the science has progressed rapidly since the separate effects of the Positive and Negative magnetic fields on biological systems were discovered in the 1930's. Used as a diagnostic, healing, and health maintenance tool, Biomagnetism has shown tremendous success in energizing the body to help relieve pain and heal many health problems. Burns, cancer, osteoarthritis, gland and organ dysfunction, rheumatism, high blood pressure, lupus, depression, poison ivy/oak, bee and insect stings and many other conditions are just a sample of some conditions that 20th century allopathic medicine has not always been effective in treating that have been resolved successfully and quickly with Biomagnetism.

Based on the principle that the biochemical mechanisms present in the human or animal body run on minute electrical currents, one may view the body as an intricate battery made up of a matrix of billions cells, all of which are essentially small living magnetic batteries. These cells form chains of intricate, interconnected circuits (tissue). When the "human battery" is fully charged and the body is healthy, these cells are properly energized and the body's electrical and cellular matrix is working properly. However, when this battery is not fully charged and/or the cells/tissue has been stressed or traumatized, their voltage has been reduced and the electro/bio/chemical matrix goes out of balance. Then normal metabolic and immune functions cannot operate efficiently, resulting in pain, inflammation, fatigue, dysfunction, possible illness and disease.

Normally at birth, and for many years thereafter, our human battery operates at full charge giving us the natural vitality necessary for a healthy life. Throughout life, the impact of physical traumas, stress, toxic exposures such as environmental pollutants, heredity, premature or normal aging can also lower the charge of the human battery and its cells which can result in illness. The term for this low-charged human battery is Magnetic Deficiency Syndrome (MDS).

Consider what happens when the battery in your car wears down: the lights dim, the circuits go into a weakened disorder and the engine will not operate correctly. The same thing happens to your body when your human battery wears down. MDS results in feeling poorly, usually accompanied by reduction of cellular functions and a gradual organ and/or gland dysfunction. Over a period of time, these metabolic dysfunctions result in further impairment of the immune system, causing incomplete healing and overall poor health.

The science of Biomagnetism is very simple. Proper use of Biomagnetism restores the healthy charge into the cells of the body which supports rapid progress toward a correction of metabolic and immune dysfunction resulting in healing and homeostasis. Biomagnetism literally RECHARGES THE HUMAN BATTERY, relieving the magnetic deficiency. Applying the proper energy field raises the lowered, insufficient electrical voltage of the body or the specific site to a normal, healthy charged voltage known as the correct zeta potential. The magnetic field's energy literally corrects the electro/bio/chemical activity by charging (exciting) the electrons of the cells to achieve their normal healthy charge resulting in the cell's metabolic and immune functions operating properly. This helps rapidly heal and reduce pain in any affected area.

As a result, at-site and systemic cellular electrical circuits and nerve transmission (neurotransmission) adjust and normalize, resulting in wellness and a return to health (homeostasis). Since Bio-Negative energy immediately neutralizes and reduces the Positive energy of inflammation, it provides excellent results in arresting pain from injury or illness. Additionally, the majority of our cases who have suffered long-term chronic conditions have shown remarkable recoveries from very basic Biomagnetic therapies.

Summary

The science of Biomagnetics is simple: The biochemical mechanisms present in the human body can be viewed as a matrix of billions of cells that run on minute electrical currents. When the cells of the human battery are charged, the body's electrical and therefore metabolism are working properly. Biomagnetism increases the body's natural energy system. When the body's vitality is low, it can be elevated Biomagnetically to help quickly resolve most painful medical conditions, illnesses, and disease.

For further information and research, see
www.BiomagScience.Net.

CHAPTER FOUR

"PLAYING WITH FIRE"

The Body Electric

Biomagnetism is the science where specifically designed magnets and their energy fields are used to affect the living system – the human body, or what has been called the "Body Electric."

There are some basic physical laws that come into play with the Body Electric. The Body Electric is the energy flow found in the human body. This energy flow is the collective result of minute electrical currents and cellular charge values that run all the functions of the cells and the body. Biomagnetism can change and elevate the electrical currents and charges – thereby increasing and maintaining the metabolic efficiency of the body's functions for health and wellness.

Magnetism, the Parent of Electricity

Our contemporary age of technology is made possible by running wires through magnetic fields to create the electricity for our homes, transportation and most things we use in everyday life. The primary physical law of magnetism is that one pole of the magnet energizes (excites) and makes all the electrons of any material in its field spin in a specific direction. The opposite pole makes the electrons spin in the opposite direction. Depending on

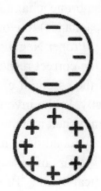

which pole is used to energize the electron spin, the charge given off will either be Positive or Negative.

Science has identified that the healthy cells have an alkaline Negative, millivoltage charge. When trauma or stress occurs, the cell changes from its healthy Negatively charged voltage to a lower Negative or Positively charged, inflamed acid-forming charge. When this occurs, the cells send an ascending signal to the brain, which computes and sends a descending return signal to flood the traumatized injured site with Negative energy to overcome and heal the traumatized, chaotic Positive charged cellular disorientation.

If the problem is acute or chronic, the tissue forms a general disorientation of very weak Negative cellular charges, or in a severely acute condition – a constant Positively-charged acid state. In this unhealthy electrical cellular climate, the cell's membrane and cytoplasm form inverse, incorrect charges, which prevent oxygen and essential micro-nutrients from entering and correctly metabolizing in the cell and prevent thorough detoxification. If this condition continues for a period of time, it leads to cellular damage, often changing the DNA, which creates many problems, including tumors.

It is important to understand that health is determined by the cell's Negative electromotive vitality for maintaining the proper electro-chemical balance, in order to maintain healthy and efficient metabolism and immune function. Cells also transfer necessary elements and spent energy (waste) electromagnetically through various membrane channels that depend on the proper energy (parallel capacitance) to work efficiently.

Proper Negative electrical vitality of the cell is also fundamental to the correct response from the DNA so that it continues to arrange all the essential elements to properly organize and metabolize correctly. In the inverse, the energy-deficient, weak-charged cells have diminished metabolic and immune functions leading to various poor health conditions resulting in illness and bad health.

Years of research and application have confirmed that the geological North, Bio-Negative magnetic energy used in a properly designed field will, in most health conditions, dynamically assist the body in rapid healing and pain relief. Increasing the healthy Negative energy to the cells helps neutralize the Positive charges of cellular inflammation from stress, trauma, injury, illness, and oxidation [by free-radicals]. Increasing the energy of low-voltage dysfunctional cells increases their health and vitality by correctly energizing their metabolism, which helps normalize immune and metabolic dysfunctions from the former sick cells.

At the atomic level, the Bio-Negative magnetic energy correctly charges (excites) the electron's energy and spin potential of the atoms of the molecules making up the cells, resulting in correctly elevating the cell's voltage and its natural ionic forces required for a healthy metabolism.

In summation, the Bio-Negative field is used in most magnet healing therapies and supports rapid pain relief and healing. It is important to note that when placing the Negative energy on any part of the limbs or shoulders, it must be placed on the proper Negative polarity meridian (see p. 103); placing the Negative energy for tissue therapy on a Positive meridian can cause stress and restrict healing.

The Bio-Positive field is generally used with the Bio-Negative field in very specific Circuit Therapies such as the MET (Meridian Energizing Therapy) or Vortex Initiation Circuit Therapies, to assist in regeneration of connective tissue, hard and soft tissue including severed nerves and nerve pathway revitalization (see "Nerve Regeneration and Meridian Energy Therapy") and to help rejoin and rapidly heal fractured or broken bones (see "fracture," Chapter 18, p. 149).

The Bio-Positive field therapy is also used to rapidly stimulate hypo gland or organ functions, as shown in "Magnetodiagnostics" (p. 83), help neutralize acid for stomachaches , help specific gastrointestinal therapies such as constipation, and help reduce pain by increasing intra- and extra-cellular fluids in the tissue in the spine when used with the Bio-Negative advanced back pain therapy.

The Bio-Negative pole therapy can be used almost any time without problems. But with the Bio-Positive field, you may be playing with fire and you must know what you are doing!

It is simple. Since normal healthy tissue has an inherent Negative charge value, it is proper to use the Bio-Negative charge to support pain relief and healing. Unless a Circuit Therapy is being used to regenerate severed or missing tissue, the use of Bio-Positive energy to charge any stressed or traumatized tissue will further stress the area, preventing it from healing properly. See Chapter Five for further discussion of the physiological effects of the different polarities.

For further information and research, see
www.BiomagScience.Net

CHAPTER FIVE

BE PRODUCT-WISE

WARNING

The Negative Pole Gives One Effect And
The Positive Pole Gives Another

Why do we give this warning? A recurrent problem in this science and in the biomagnetic health and research industry is that magnet manufacturers, and many people in general, do not understand the important difference in universally marking the poles correctly. Additionally, many companies selling biomagnets are ignorant about the proper application of field therapies and what is the correct field of a medical magnet.

It is very important for you to understand the basic, vital difference between the geological North (Negative) and South (Positive) Pole effects and to be 'product-wise' when selecting magnetic products to be used for health therapies.

For example: Many magnet manufacturers put an 'N' or an 'S' on their magnets. But their 'N' or 'S' marking is an engineer's symbol and means North- or South-seeking pole. What seeks the North? The South seeks the North. That means the 'N' on the magnet may be the South (Positive) Pole, a dangerous pole to use indiscriminately!

This is important because using incorrectly marked magnets can be very dangerous to your health, such as if you apply an N-marked magnet thinking it was the Geo North Pole when it is the North seeking Bio-Positive energy field, that can charge the weak cells into a Positive cancerous state. Knowledgeable biomagnetic scientists and practitioners agree: it is of the utmost importance that biomagnetic applications are very specific and accurate in applying the proper energy fields and that medical magnets should uniformly be electromotively marked Negative (-) and Positive (+) to ensure the correct energy for the application.

Based on the simple laws of physics, the wrong side of the magnet placed over sensitive tissue can cause inflammation and stress, which can lead to damaging your health. Remember, as outlined in the previous chapter, South Pole is Positive. Positive is stimulating and stimulates all forms of life including bacteria, viruses, inflammation, cancer cell growth rates, etc.

The geological North Pole is Negative. Negative charges create Negative energy, the body's natural calming, healing energy.

These are polarity charges of the geological North and South Poles of the earth and a magnet:

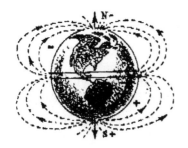 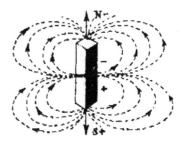

Since most people do not know the difference between the true poles and the "seeking" poles of a magnet, BiomagScience has chosen to use the universal healing color green and its Negative (-) marking for the Bio-Negative side of its medical magnets, and the universal color red and its Positive (+) marking for the Bio-Positive side of its medical magnets. For your safety, all BiomagScience medical magnets (BioMagnets) are triple tested with a measuring instrument known as a magnetometer. This testing device accurately reads Negative (geological North) and Positive (geological South).

Be aware of what kind of biomagnets you're getting before you buy. Insist on true geological North (Negative) and South (Positive).

Remember that wrong pole markings can be very harmful to your health.

Polarity Test for Magnets

To test magnets for correct polarity, you'll need a compass. The needle of the compass that points to the geological North Pole of the earth will point to the true Bio-Negative North Pole of the magnet (and vice versa).

Some commercially marketed magnetic products are produced by business people who do not understand the basic scientific principles of biomagnetic science. Unfortunately, these products are not as easy to test. Such a product is the Multi-Polar Pad. Again, Buyer Beware! Using this kind of magnetic device can be a costly mistake for your health.

Multi-Polar Pads and Your Health
WARNING

This, below, is a magnetic pad worn on the body. It varies in size from credit card-sized to as big as 9" by 12" or larger and has alternating North/South, Negative/Positive, multi-polar magnetic fields in varying designs.

| N | S | N | S | N | S | N | S |

Knowledgeable researchers worldwide are shocked about these systems! Using this type of magnetic field just applied anywhere on the body without proper guidelines is like giving a child a medical kit with a scalpel and saying, "Okay, you're a surgeon now, go out and practice. You've got your Doctorate!"

The multi-pole magnetic pad has multiple charges.
What exactly does this mean in terms of health?

Scientific measurement of the alternating Negative/Positive configuration magnetic fields in a multi-polar pad indicates an aggregate (or sum) of 7%-14% Positive Geo South pole energy is being emitted from the pad.

In understanding why a multi-polar pad emits an aggregate or sum of Bio-Positive energy, consider light and dark. If you mix both of them, you will get light although it won't be as bright. The Positive is stimulating expanding (light) and the Negative is calming contracting (dark). Since the Positive energy is expanding, it will always be larger than the Negative. That is why when both poles are mixed in the aggregate, the sum of both puts out Bio-Positive energy. Remember, most healing requires amplifying the Negative healing energy of the body, not the acid- and inflammation-producing Bio-Positive energy.

Upon first usage, the multi-polar biomagnet often makes one feel better, as the Bio-Positive stimulates the metabolism, just the way a cup of coffee makes one feel good because it speeds up the system. Not that this is a good idea, because at the cellular level, prolonged Positive stimulation of the metabolism and cellular tissue promotes acidosis, inflammation, increases free-radical site damage, increases dysfunction of the cells and immune system, and reduces transport efficiency of oxygen, nutrition and detoxification – all leading to illness and disease.

The multi-polar configuration stresses the body with Positive charges that signals the brain to transmit more Negative energy to relieve the stress. This is analogous to putting a lit match to a burn to make it heal faster. The continued stimulation of stress can lead to aberrant growth behavior where the cells weaken, lose their charge, go into a Positive acid state and start to mutate. Furthermore, prolonged use of the multi-polar therapy will start to influence and weaken the healthy Negative charged surrounding tissue and start to spread throughout the body. As a result, the entire body can lose its healthy electromotive vitality and start to spiral downward into acidosis, illness and disease.

To reiterate, in the body's natural healing mode, when an area is traumatized or stressed, the cells become disoriented, chaotic, and inflamed with their charge going into a low Negative and/or Positive state which signals the brain to send healing Negative charges to the site. The disoriented sick cells and tissue naturally, electromagnetically absorb the healing Negative energy until they normalize into their balanced, healthy Negatively charged state. At that point, the brain stops sending healing Negative energy to the site.

An example of the Bio-Positive reactions is the case of a middle-aged woman who had to have someone with her during waking hours because she was so suicidal from constant overwhelming pain. We searched and found that she had an extremely expensive multi-polar bed from Japan that was creating unremitting inflammation in her body. We suggested getting rid of the bed and as soon as she did, the pain and inflammation went away. Then she used BiomagScience Daytime therapy and bio-energized Negative water and got her vitality and health back very quickly.

These types of type multi-polar mattresses and pads have been shown to debilitate individuals, giving them fibromyalgia, CFS, Candida and many other conditions due to the excess of the Bio-Positive energy which stimulates inflammation and dysfunction of the metabolism and immune system.

If the cells are sick (low charged) for a long period, perhaps from the influence of an external source of Bio-Positive energy from EMF or a multi-polar therapy pad, their cytoplasm can lose its Negative voltage entirely and go into a Positive state, which produces lactic acid, moving the cell from normal functioning to metabolizing sugar as its primary nutrient. This can stop apoptosis (normal cellular death), as the Positively charged DNA starts replicating the aberrant cells, creating tumors and cancer. Here is a rather simple analogy: doctors prescribe ice to reduce inflammation and swelling, not heat.

Like ice, the Bio-Negative field is calming, healing and helps reduce inflammation and swelling. The Positive field, like heat, is stimulating and therefore increases inflammation and swelling.

Multi-polar companies warn not to use their products for kidney disease, viral or bacterial problems, cancer, sinusitis and other ailments. What this really means is, **MULTI-POLAR MAGNETS ARE BAD FOR YOUR HEALTH.** Medical magnets work well on these conditions.

It is important to note that besides MET (Meridian Energizing Therapy) for systemically energizing and balancing the body's biochemistry and Circuit Therapy for initiating healing and regeneration of tissue, there are a few areas of the body where it is recommended that application of Bio-Positive energy be done concurrently with Daytime or CVS therapy in order to maintain overall cellular health.

1. **Back Pain:** Often caused by muscle weakness or trauma, the Bio-Positive pole on the spine in conjunction with the two Bio-Negative side applications increases the inter- and intracellular fluids in the tissue of the spine. This expands and separates the vertebrae which helps stop the nerve pinching and its pain. Case studies show that the Back Circuit Therapy of the Positive pole used in conjunction with two-side Negative poles provides fast pain relief and helps heal the affected tissue, thereby reducing the likelihood that the condition will return.

   Note: It is important to use the Daytime (sternum) or CVS therapy at the same time in order to ensure that the body is maintaining the correct charge. (See "Back, Sciatica Therapy" and ♥PD Warning.)

2. **Acid indigestion** of the stomach: The Bio-Positive energy placed over the stomach helps relieve acid indigestion. However, a glass of Bio-Negative energized water also provides very quick relief of acid indigestion.

3. **Digestion aid / Constipation:** Apply the Bio-Positive energy over the center of the groin for 10-15 minutes after eating to aid digestion and peristalsis – the muscular action of the colon. The same therapy also helps overcome constipation. See Chapters 14 and 15 for therapies.

Summary

The Bio-Negative and specialized Bio-Positive field Circuit Therapies on the body can be critical to any success in health, and when used properly, have shown no contraindications (bad side effects). Remember that Bio-Negative therapy can be used almost any time without causing a problem. However, with the Bio-Positive field, you must know what you are doing!

Beware of multi-polar systems and remember to wear the Daytime or applicable CVS application during any Bio-Positive therapy to maintain the correct healthy body charge.

For further information and research, see
www.BiomagScience.Net

It is important to note that all therapies must be handled with care. Please refer to "Precautions," Chapter 15 for certain restrictions in the application of magnets.

CHAPTER SIX

THE TRUTH ABOUT MAGNET POWER

Worldwide, biomagnetic researchers have consistently shown that the more powerful the bio-magnet, the deeper it penetrates into the tissue and the faster it relieves the pain and helps the body heal.

Size and material composition are the most important factors regulating the power and the healing properties of a magnet. Bio-Magnets from BiomagScience are made from the most powerful magnetic ore in the world, known as Rare Earth Neodymium iron. Recognized in the late twentieth century for its powerful magnetic properties, Rare Earth gave us a biomagnetic power breakthrough.

Before the new advanced Rare Earth Super Magnet technology was introduced, biomagnets had to be large and cumbersome to provide the necessary therapy power. But even the huge and heavy 5-6 pound 4"x6"x1" thick ceramic magnet cannot penetrate the body as effectively as the much easier to apply BiomagScience Super Bio-magnet, which has almost three times the power, is 1/50th the size, and weighs about an ounce.

First, it is important to understand how a magnet is rated. Magnets are measured in units of gauss (pronounced "gows"). Gauss is a unit of measurement which defines how many lines of magnetic force (flux) per square centimeter are emitted from the surface of the pole of the magnet.

Today, while there has been the power breakthrough with Rare Earth Super magnets, many biomagnet sellers remain ignorant in rating their biomagnets. Instead of providing the *true surface gauss,* they use the internal rating known as the *br. Coersive,* which is the power it takes to magnetize or demagnetize the particular magnet composition.

The *br. Coersive* and its Oerstedt measurement along with the thickness, size and shape is what determines the surface gauss, which determines the width and depth of penetration of useful flux therapy energy. For example, a number of sellers state their biomagnets have 14,800 gauss, but do not supply the surface reading which indicates how deep and wide the biomagnets will penetrate the tissue and for what kind of therapy it is effective.

A 14,000 gauss internal field can produce 200, 500, 2000, 2500, 3000, 3500 or more surface gauss. If a seller states only the internal 14,800 gauss and not the surface gauss, they do not know the basics of magnetism and cannot be trusted to know the proper difference between the North or South or Negative or Positive or the proper strength of their medical magnets for the therapy to be addressed. Buyer beware! These improperly marked magnets could be *very dangerous* to your health.

BiomagScience BioMagnets are made from the new, breakthrough, rare-earth Super magnets. They are extremely powerful and have replaced all the old fashioned magnets most practitioners have used before. All BiomagScience magnets are Super BioMagnets and are calibrated for the proper tissue penetration, which is essential when the correct healing support is required.

An example of the new breakthrough is the easy-to-wear BiomagScience's Super BioMagnet, which is 1.25" in diameter, 0.75" thick and weighs only a couple of ounces. About 1/50th the size, it replaces the 6 lb 4"x6"x1" ceramic therapy magnets used by many practitioners and provides deeper penetration than the huge ceramic magnets. An example of using the Super BioMagnet is energizing the liver, where the condition requires deep and wide field penetration. The magnet can easily be worn all day and night while providing better therapy than the cumbersome huge ceramic magnet.

BiomagScience's Power Wafers and Regulars are even smaller and can easily be applied and used at all times. Like the Super, their energy is specifically designed for whatever the therapy requires to address the particular condition.

Summary

Insist on true North (-) and South (+) magnets. Know what strength magnet is needed for the therapies you'll be using. For deep tissue therapy such as organ, gland, bone, cartilage, etc., it is important to use biomagnets that are scientifically designed for proper tissue penetration.

BEWARE of companies that offer high gauss magnets, such as 14,800G (gauss) without also stating the surface gauss; you should be wary about buying them, as you may be getting improperly marked magnets without the power to do the therapy. And if the company offers therapy guidance, they may be ignorant about the actual science, which means that you could be hurt.

Always make sure you are getting certified medical magnets that are specifically designed for the correct depth of penetration for the specific therapy. Otherwise, you are playing with fire. Biomag-Science BioMagnets have been specially designed for their required penetration values and are certified as medical magnets by the Foundation for Magnetic Sciences. This author respectfully suggests that you use them.

BIOMAGNETIC POWER RATINGS

Dates retested: January 2012, 2013, 2014, 2015, 2016
Meter: AlphaLab Model GM-1-ST Certification of Calibration Serial # 596, ISO/IEC 17025:2005 ANSI/NCSL Z4540-1-1994

Gauss: Surface; Primary & Secondary Active Field Depth/Width Measurements

BiomagScience Biomagnetic Power Values since 2007

Model	Width & Penetration Depth	Bio-Negative Surface Gauss	Primary Field Depth & Width	Secondary Field Strength
Power Wafer (PW)	Topical Lite	2020	1"d x 1.5" w	3.25"d x 3.5" w
2-Stack PW	Lite Med Wide/Deep	2600	1.5"d x 2.5"w	4"d x 4"w
Regular (R)	Medium Wide/Deep	2300	2.5"d x 2.5"w	8"d x 5"w
2-Stack R*	Very Wide/Deep	2780	3.5"d x 5"w	18"d x 6"w
Super	Very, Very Wide/Deep	3150	5"d x 6"w	22"d x 7.5w

BiomagScience 2-Stack* of Regulars has a strong secondary field penetration of 20 inches. A single Super** BioMagnet has a strong secondary Gama field penetration of 22 inches for extremely deep tissue therapy.

BMI Single Pole Biomagnets
Negative Side (only)   **Average-300**

Homedics TheraP–Bi Polar   **Average-600**

Nikken Bi-Polar– "Bio Mini"
+/– Majority Area Reading   **20**
+/– Edge Reading   **70**

CHAPTER SEVEN

MAGNETIZED
STRUCTURED WATER

Through the years, people who drink energized, structured water consistently report feeling better. Aches and pains are reported to go away along with many conditions such as kidney stones, gallstones, arthritis, high-blood pressure, fatigue and other uncomfortable problems. The question is, why does energized structured water affect and increase the body's health? What is it about the Bio-Negatively charged structured water from Lourdes, France or Hunza Pakistan that creates the miracle healing and vitality?

When water enters the body, a certain amount of its molecules are separated by a special hormone into their hydrogen and oxygen atoms which the body uses independently. Oxygen supports cellular metabolic and immune functions and helps detoxify cellular waste (spent energy) while the hydrogen [ions] are the first basic electrical component in the proper functioning of glands and organs.

The function of the hydrogen ion is shown in Magneto-Diagnostics where a testing magnet is used over each gland or organ to test whether it has the proper amount of hydrogen activity. If it is low in hydrogen, there is a reflexive response to the Negative pole, indicating a hypo-hydrogen state. Most unhealthy low or dysfunctioning organ or glandular conditions are shown to have a hypo-hydrogen condition, indicating the body is low in hydrogen. Although rare, if there is a response to the Positive pole, the body has too much hydrogen, indicating a hyper-hydrogen state (see "Magneto-Diagnostics").

Although the body receives most of its oxygen from breathing, it receives most of its hydrogen from water. This is another important reason that drinking enough water daily is recommended, in order for your body to get its proper amount of hydrogen.

In all liquid chemistry, molecules of the same type cluster together like a bunch of grapes, in what is known as chemical associations.

When these normal molecular water clusters enter your body after drinking a glass of water, only the outer molecules of the clusters can metabolize with the hormone because the hormone cannot access the interior molecules of the cluster. This results in a lack of proper hydrogen in the glands and organs. Over a period of time and often manifesting in middle age, the lack of hydrogen ions in the glands and organs starts to take a toll of not being able to operate efficiently, often resulting first in fatigue and then in illness and/or disease.

In addition, because of their size, these naturally occurring molecular water clusters cannot efficiently hydrate the cells, and as a result, there is a reduction of nutrition and oxygen transfer into the cells and detoxification out of the cells, further preventing the cells from maintaining a healthy state.

Bio-Energizing Water

Since water molecules are comprised of atoms which all have electrons, the electrons can be energized with a magnetic field. When water is magnetically energized, all the electrons take on the same charge. Because like-charges repel, the molecules are forced away from each other, breaking up the clusters into single molecules *(monatomic molecules)* and micro-clusters.

When the energized monatomic water molecules enter the body, more of the molecules can be accessed and metabolized by the hormone that naturally separates the oxygen and hydrogen. As a result, there is an increase of hydrogen ion availability, which supplements and resolves the hypo-hydrogen gland/organ condition resulting in normalizing the gland/organ functions. Another key benefit of the small-sized single molecules of monatomic water is the increase in cellular transport efficiency. There is literally increased cell hydration, increased oxygen and nutrition going into the cells, and greater detoxification out of the cells, all of which increase health and vitality.

In the famed Lourdes and Hunza water, a geological structure naturally energizes the water and is the reason why people drinking it experience an increase in wellness. By the same token, drinking energized water every day will produce an increase in wellness daily.

Many people who use a magnetic water softener have reported that they feel better, have better skin tone, and feel an overall increase in health. When learning about the health benefits of energized water, they often inquire whether they should drink Negatively or Positively charged water, because both charges break up the clusters into energized monatomic water molecules.

Years of application and research indicate that specifically for health purposes, *Bio-Negative energized structured water is preferred* as it provides additional healthy Negative energy to the body, thus supporting and promoting wellness much more rapidly.

BiomagScience makes *Water Jar Energizers* for the home and travel and the *Under-the-Sink Negative Energizer* for a continuous flow of healthy Bio-Negatively charged structured water.

As it is so effective in helping increase health and support rapid healing, Bio-Negative energized water is used in most therapies in this book. This water is also highly useful to help heal burns, scrapes and upset stomachs. If you have a stomachache, a glass of Bio-Negative energized water will help immediately resolve it. If a person feels nervous and upset, a glassful will help relax him or her immediately.

Clinical results have indicated Bio-Negative energized water used in conjunction with the lower CVS Bio-Negative field therapy has positive results in people with Alzheimer's disease.

When Bio-Negative charged water is combined with BAO (See BiomagScience Activated Oxygen, in the next chapter), using it internally becomes an amazing formula for quickly increasing blood oxygen levels for a rapid increase in energy. Using the combination externally, it provides rapid relief from poison ivy/oak and immediate therapy for burns, as it hydrates the burned skin, delivering oxygen where normal water cannot.

Summary

Case studies and long term research have shown conclusively that Bio-Negative energized water supplementation has healing powers.

Internal: Bio-Negative energized structured water increases natural energy in the body. Drink this water daily for general wellness. And it is especially effective with most therapies for supportive healing. For a rapid increase in energy within ten minutes, add BAO (See "BiomagScience Activated Oxygen," in the next chapter) to a glass of Bio-Negative Energized Structured Water.

External: Bio-Negative Energized Structured Water and BAO combined has also shown extraordinary, rapid healing powers when used as an immediate therapy for skin conditions such as poison ivy/oak, psoriasis, acne, burns, bedsores, melanoma, cuts and scrapes.

For product information and research, see p. 241.
www.BiomagScience.Net.

CHAPTER EIGHT

IMPORTANCE OF ACTIVATED OXYGEN

It is known by medical science that a lack of oxygen at a cellular level is the main problem behind many illnesses and diseases. Oxygen is the metabolizing and detoxifying agent of the body. All human cellular tissue needs oxygen to function.

Oxygen Functions to:

1. Catalyze cellular constituents for metabolism and energy production.

2. Stimulate the growth and development of normal, beneficial bacteria (aerobic).

3. Kill viruses and infectious (anaerobic) bacteria.

4. Detoxify cellular tissue by removing waste via the circulatory system; carbon dioxide is transported in the blood to the lungs where an exchange of large quantities of oxygen and carbon dioxide takes place.

In addition to the fact that there is a general depletion of oxygen in the atmosphere, poor diet, inadequate exercise, environmental toxins, and emotional and physical stress also contribute toward an acid condition in the body. More oxygen is then required to help neutralize the acidity, and without enough oxygen, premature aging and bad health can occur – a vicious cycle.

Have you ever seen a runner gasping for air at the end of the race? The athletic term "oxygen debt" was coined to describe the inadequate amount of oxygen to oxygenate and remove the lactic acid that high-energy athletic exertion creates. In other words, oxygen deprivation is natural in sports. People who are out of shape gasp for air after minimal exercise due to a lack of lung function to provide enough oxygen. People also feel invigorated after getting a breath of fresh air outside after leaving a stuffy room.

When individuals are very ill, the first thing they receive in the hospital is pure oxygen. Oxygen deprivation is one of the main causes of a weakened immune system. Increased oxygenation strengthens the immune system. It is not hard to understand how important oxygen is.

Hydrogen Peroxide

Hydrogen peroxide (H_2O_2) has been used for decades on cuts or burns to immediately help stop germs. The reason it is so effective is that it contains the active germicide, oxygen. Pure hydrogen peroxide has also been used in drinking water for increasing the body's oxygen levels. After drinking H_2O_2, heart and emphysema patients are able to walk further distances or climb stairs without gasping for air.

The major problem with H_2O_2 is that it is very unstable and can produce a Super Free Radical – a highly unstable, Positive molecule that immediately bonds and destroys healthy tissue, if the H_2O_2 is taken when the stomach is not entirely empty. It has been shown that within a couple of weeks of improperly taking H_2O_2 with food that contains any iron, the super free radicals can create stomach cancer. Therefore, H_2O_2 is not considered the safest form of oxygen.

BiomagScience Activated Oxygen

BiomagScience Activated Oxygen (BAO) uses an advanced formula that produces a safe, liquid-oxygen that increases the blood oxygen percentage. This, in turn, increases energy, metabolic and immune functions, and helps the body kill infectious (anaerobic) bacteria. Unlike drugs and antibiotics, it does not harm the beneficial (aerobic) bacteria.

What is BiomagScience Activated Oxygen (BAO)?

BAO is a nontoxic, aqueous solution of various oxides of chlorites with a high concentration of oxygen in stable molecular form developed with additional donor electrons so that while being used in the body, if any of its electrons are naturally stripped from the oxygen molecule, there are always enough to maintain stability in providing oxygen to the body without becoming an oxide (oxidant – super free radical). The oxygen molecules are absorbed into the bloodstream and travel via the red blood cells throughout the body to assist in cellular metabolism, energy production and waste elimination.

BAO is a safe form of oxygen to take for elevating the body's oxygen level. While increased oxygen increases vitality in cellular metabolism, it also selectively kills harmful, anaerobic infectious bacteria.

BAO cannot over-oxidize the cells because the iron atoms (in the red blood cells) only release the amount of oxygen that the cell can utilize.

BAO is an oxygen in liquid concentrate that does not dissipate, nor will it dissipate when ingested or added to other liquids. It is non-caloric and absolutely safe.

BAO is effective against all anaerobic bacteria: Salmonella, cholera, E. coli, pneumonia, streptococcus, Pseudomonas, Staphylococcus, Giardia lamblia and various microorganisms. Nothing unfavorable in the body can live very long in an oxygen-rich environment.

As an example, the yeast Candida albicans is normal in small quantities in the intestines. When the oxygen level in the body is low, acidity increases, and as a result, the yeast (Candida) increases, producing large quantities that become toxic. Candida reduces the immune system's ability to fend off disease and illness and also reduces the ability of the liver and other organs to function properly.

Treating Candida with BAO, Energized Negative Water, and Negative BioMagnetic Therapy helps to immediately change the acidic condition to alkaline, which creates an unfriendly electro/bio/chemical terrain for the yeast to thrive, thus creating a friendly environment for health.

The range of applications for using BAO include arthritis, asthma/breathing, heart attacks, bronchitis, bed sores, burns, candidiasis, colds, cold sores, cuts, cirrhosis, colitis, diarrhea, dysentery, emphysema, fever blisters, food poisoning, fungi, protozoa, parasites, gangrene, hay fever, indigestion, infection, joint pain, poison ivy/oak, seizures, and sunburn.

Another example is the individual who, with pneumonia, was breathing very hard yet could not get enough oxygen in his lungs, with the result that he felt he was suffocating. He immediately took a strong dose of BAO in water and within minutes was able to relax his breathing because his blood oxygen level went up enough to satisfy his need.

Questions and Answers about BAO

Q: What does oxygen do?
A: Oxygen is the source of life and energy to all cells. At a cellular level, oxygen is more than just something we breathe. Every cell in our body is like a little organ with a specific job to do; it needs oxygen to do the job properly. Known as cellular respiration, oxygen works to carry the needed nutrients to the cell, produce energy inside the cell, and then remove waste products from the cell.

Without sufficient oxygen in our system to support the health of the cells, they lose their energy, acidify and use sugar fermentation as their source of energy. This causes a breakdown of the entire cellular chemistry and adversely affects the body's immune system's ability to operate correctly.

Q: What happens if I don't get enough oxygen?
A: Lack of oxygen is one of the leading causes of disease and illness. Insufficient oxygen due to stress, poor nutrition, lack of exercise and air pollution can result in anything from general fatigue to serious illness. Many diseases, including cancer, are linked to insufficient oxygen.

Q: Don't I get enough oxygen from breathing?
A: What used to be is no longer true. Due to deforestation and the toxic contaminants of our industrialized society, the oxygen levels in the earth's atmosphere are much lower. The air in which most people grew up used to be a minimum of 20% oxygen. In Japan and other populated cities worldwide, the oxygen level has dropped to 12% and in some cities, it is much less. If you need to increase the oxygen in your system, BAO is an easy and excellent method, and when used with Bio-Negative energized structured water, the increase in oxygen ion availability can help normalize your blood oxygen percentage. Just try it; you will love the increased energy.

Q: What does BAO do?
A: BAO provides more oxygen to your physiological system. Adding oxygen to your body helps the oxygen functions in the body. BAO is nontoxic and destroys harmful bacteria without harming beneficial bacteria. As a solution of stabilized electrolytes of oxygen in molecular form, it can also purify the water we drink and kill all types of anaerobic infectious bacteria while stimulating the beneficial bacteria internally.

Q: How does BAO work?
A: When BAO is taken, it is absorbed through the digestive process and distributed throughout the body via the circulatory system for cellular respiration and metabolic functions.

Q: What are the benefits?
A: Anaerobic (bad) bacteria, viruses and unfriendly micro-organisms are unable to survive in the presence of oxygen. The immune system works to repair physical damage resulting from stressful conditions, such as infections, toxic chemicals, free-radicals, and physical trauma, but it depends on oxygen and the ability of the body's cells to metabolize properly.

BAO is especially noted for its nontoxic, antibacterial properties. It helps improve immune functions. It is a beneficial therapy for Candida, cirrhosis of the liver, colitis, Crohn's disease, emphysema, food poisoning, fungus, gangrene, indigestion, poison ivy/oak, polyps, Raynaud's disease, skin cancer, burns and most medical conditions. (See chapter on BioMagnetic Therapies.)

Q: How is it taken?
A: For internal use, it is suggested to take BAO diluted in drinking water. Just put the correct amount of drops in a glass of Energized Negative Water and drink. (See BAO Dosage, p. 53.) When using externally for burns, insect bites and other skin care problems, simply mix BAO in a smaller amount of Bio-Negative Energized Water. It can also be used to purify drinking water and washing your food with this solution will decontaminate it.

Q: How often do you take BAO?
A: Drinking two to three glasses of BAO with Energized Negative Water daily is an excellent way to elevate oxygen levels, increase vitality, and fight off infectious bacteria in the body.

Q: Can BAO really make my water safe to drink?
A: BAO kills coliform bad bacteria and microorganisms in water. Laboratory reports show 10 drops of BAO in 8 oz. of mountain water kills the organism Giardia lamblia, in just 2 1/2 minutes.

Q: Will this product give me more energy?
A: Definitely! BAO supplies oxygen in molecular form to the body. Athletes report they have more energy and stamina after using 20 drops in water or juice 3 times daily.

Q: Can I overdose with BAO?
A: Yes, but it is unusual. BAO is nontoxic and will give a slight stomach ache or a minor case of diarrhea if you take a lot more than the recommended dosage. If you get a stomach ache, immediately drink a glass of Energized Negative Water and you will feel better.

Q: Should I refrigerate BAO?
A: No. Although the government label laws state that supplements cannot have a shelf life of over two years, BAO has been shown to have an indefinite shelf life. Keep a bottle at home, in your car, when you travel and in your First-Aid kit. It is advised to keep it away from direct sunlight.

Typical BAO Therapy Testimonials

Heart Problem: Oxygen is helpful to people with heart problems. A Malaysian man in his mid-sixties had a heart condition with only a 30% blood flow and was very low in energy. He could not afford the surgery and his doctor was surprised he did not have a heart attack, but told him to continue to do whatever he was doing since no necrosis had set in. He continued drinking BAO in energized water 5 times daily along with keeping a Bio-Negative Energy magnet over his heart. He was able to sustain his strength for over 3 months before having a successful by-pass surgery.

Poison Oak: A friend called me after hiking in the woods on a warm day. She had contracted a major case of poison oak that covered both her legs with a livid-red itchy rash. I told her to spray the affected area with a solution of 50 drops BAO per 2 oz. of Bio-Negative Energized Water. She called back an hour later saying, "It's all gone."

Walking Pneumonia was the diagnosis. Our production manager had just returned from the doctor's office and was on her way home for two weeks of bed rest. I instructed her to take 50 drops of BAO in 8 oz. of water every 4 hours and reduce the dosage to 40 drops the next day. I told her we would see her when she was better. To my surprise, she was at work the very next morning. The pneumonia was gone overnight.

People who travel can conveniently treat their drinking water with BAO to kill bacteria and other micro-organisms. Likewise, travelers can also wash their vegetables with it to make sure they don't get sick from E coli.

A note from the author

A number of years ago, I was working on my motorcycle and the gas tank exploded. Second-degree burns spanned the entire length of my right arm from the fingertips to my shoulder. Of course, this was very painful.

I was knowledgeable about both the oxygen and Negative pole water benefits, so I immediately drank Energized Negative Water with BAO (50 drops per glass) and also mixed 75 drops of BAO in 4 ounces of Bio-Negative Energized Water, which I sprayed on my arm every hour. Within moments of spraying, the pain subsided by 80% and within a short time after that, the tremendous swelling went down. I kept up the spraying and increased my electrolytes. About six days later, my skin was healed.

This made me realize how important it was to use both BAO and Energized Negative Water together. Although in most cases second-degree burns should always be treated by properly trained medical persons, BAO is a valuable First-Aid therapy that comes with the Wellness Kit and can be mixed with Bio-Negative water to produce a strong healing solution for burns.

Most therapies in this book include the use of Bio-Negative Energized Water with BAO. The healing properties of each are amplified by using them together. We have seen cases of poison ivy/ oak going away in half an hour. All burns have been shown to heal much more rapidly with low or no pain levels. Patients with arterial heart blockage were able to live in comfort for some time before their heart surgery. We have seen walking pneumonia disappear overnight, rather than after the 2 weeks the doctor indicated.

BiomagScience Activated Oxygen comes in a drop-by-drop squeeze bottle that is very easy to use for individual dosages. Each bottle has 2.33 fluid ounces or a month's daily supply. Use it on a daily basis with Energized Negative Water as an important supplement for good health, or keep a bottle in your First-Aid Kit for emergencies.

Note: Always drink 3-4 glasses a day of Bio-Energized water to avoid dehydration.

BAO DOSAGE

For Best Results:

- Use with Energized Negative Water.
- External: Do not use on eyes, ears, or nose without diluting in water – 15 drops per 1/4 cup water.
- Do not store in sunlight.
- Do not take 3-4 hours before bedtime. BAO may energize and keep you awake.

Drinking Bio-Negative Energized Water 3 Times per day:
Babies: 2 drops per small glass of water.
Small children: 3-4 drops per glass of water.
Large Children: 5-8 drops per glass of water.
Adults: 15-20 drops per glass of water.

Water Storage:
For short-term water storage, use 12 drops per gallon to prevent algae/bacterial growth. For long-term storage, use 20 drops per gallon.

Milk and Juices:
10-15 drops per quart will extend freshness up to several weeks in most cases.

Athletes and Joggers:
Use 20-30 or more drops in Bio-Negative Energized Water.

Bee Stings and Insect Bites: One drop applied to the bite.
Put a 2-Stack Negative Power Wafers immediately on the bite to stop any swelling.

Breathing Attacks/Heart Attack:
50 drops in two ounces of Bio-Negative Energized Water.
Bronchitis/Emphysema/Sinus:
Add 20-30 drops to 8 oz. Bio-Negative Energized Water, three times daily.

Fever Blisters, Cold Sores, Herpes:
Mix 30 drops of BAO in 1 oz. of Energized Negative Water and dab directly on blister or sore. For a wound or cold sores in the mouth, mix 30 drops of BAO in 2 oz. of Energized Negative Water – wash or gargle.

Food Poisoning, Dysentery/Diarrhea:
Add 25 drops to 8 oz. of juice or water. Take twice over 3 hours. For baby use 3-5 drops.

Gums, Mouth and Teeth:
5 or 6 drops on the toothbrush while brushing teeth.
5 drops in ½ oz. water for mouthwash or gargle.

Infections, Flu Virus:
At first sign, 20-30 drops of BAO in Energized Negative Water three times daily for a minimum of 3 days.

Note: For people who weigh 70-100 pounds, use 15 drops in a glass of Energized water. For a child less than 70 pounds, cut the dosage to 5-6 drops in half a glass. For babies, cut the dosage to 2 drops in a quarter of a glass.

Poison Oak/Ivy, Skin Cuts and Small Burns:
75 drops of BAO in 4 oz. Energized Negative Water. Wash and spray.

There are many more applications of this wonderful oxygen formula in the therapy section of this book.

CHAPTER NINE

NUTRITION

The Importance of Vitamins, Minerals and Diet

A leading cause of poor health is the lack of proper minerals and nutrients in our diet. In the early 1900's the U.S. Congress published an agricultural report that stated most of the essential minerals in soil had been depleted and were no longer available. Now in the 21st century, this depletion is even more pronounced and widespread. Even the purest organic crops, which are rotated and grown without pesticides, are mineral deficient and cannot produce all the vitamins and nutrients needed for good health. Organic crops may have more nutrients than traditionally grown crops, but supplementation is still indicated to achieve optimal nutrition. Therefore, it is essential to take quality nutritional supplements on a regular basis.

Vitamins and Minerals

Taking the right amount of the right kinds of vitamins, minerals, and other nutrients is not a simple task, since such a wide variety of different supplements are available. Understandably, each manufacturer would have you believe that their preparations are the best ones you can buy. The following concepts need to be considered when choosing the best supplementation.

It is absolutely vital to take vitamin and mineral supplements that most closely approach the forms in which they are found in food. Properly chelated vitamin and mineral supplements seem to best fulfill the "food form" concept. A chelated supplement is one that has the same types of molecules found in the natural breakdown or digestion of food. These food associated molecules are attached to the vitamins or minerals being given. Such "companion" molecules include amino acids, small proteins, and carbohydrates.

The primary importance of taking chelated supplements is that the bioavailability of the nutrient is optimized. Although often represented as such, bioavailability is not the same as mere absorption. Bioavailability involves the proper delivery of a nutrient to the proper tissue binding sites in the body. Absorption means only that something gets into the bloodstream. Because of this, the absorbability of a supplement can be misleading. More is not necessarily better, and is often worse.

The best sources of minerals, those found in food, will often only demonstrate a 10%-20% degree of absorption. Other forms, such as those found in colloidal organic mineral preparations, may actually have greater than 90% absorbability. However, getting an ionic form of a mineral rapidly absorbed into the blood stream is not the same as getting that mineral delivered to the target sites in the target tissues.

Properly chelated minerals and other nutrients also protect the tissues from being overwhelmed or overdosed by too much of these supplements. Too much will ultimately be as bad as too little. Proper delivery of nutrients insures that only small amounts will be required to meet the body's needs. Flooding the bloodstream with large amounts of easily absorbed mineral forms may allow the target tissue sites to receive what they need, but those mineral forms will be over-accumulating elsewhere. This over-accumulation, even of good minerals, can have its own substantial toxicity.

In other words, a highly absorbable mineral form is not necessarily a bio-available form of that mineral. Many minerals in many natural foods have a fairly limited absorption. At the very least, if you are uncertain whether a supplement is in a chelated form, steer clear of high-milligram, low-cost supplements, since they are often a variation on nothing more than ground-up rock (literally!).

Look for low-milligram (or microgram), more expensive supplements as a general rule, since these will tend to be more bio-available supplements. When they are in the right form, minerals and other nutrients are needed in only relatively small amounts.

In reference to colloidal mineral/vitamin supplements, it is important to know what additional elements are in the supplement. Even when advertised as coming from ancient plant sources, it is important to realize that ancient plant sources are no more like food than a 1000-year-old hamburger. Furthermore, plants are fairly indiscriminate in absorbing and retaining all mineral elements to which they are exposed, toxic or otherwise.

Some supplement manufacturers actually recommend plant-derived supplements that contain lead, cadmium, beryllium (one of the most carcinogenic elements known to man), mercury (the most toxic non-radioactive heavy metal known to man), and a host of other toxic mineral elements. Even in the tiniest amounts, these toxic elements can be expected to accumulate in the body over time. This means that someone may initially experience beneficial health effects from restoring levels of necessary minerals. However, toxicity will result from the long-term, regular ingestion of such colloidal mineral sources as the toxic elements continue to accumulate.

When used on a shorter-term basis and when properly purified of toxic mineral elements, colloidal mineral sources can be beneficial. However, even when purified, the high absorbability of these colloidal minerals will eventually overdose you on the "good" minerals. Remember to always read your labels and don't be afraid to ask questions when buying your supplements.

Summary

The best vitamin and mineral supplements are properly chelated forms. These supplements may sometimes come from food sources directly, or they can sometimes be synthesized in a form bound to the proper molecules.

Amino acids do not generally need supplementation if you are eating and properly digesting adequate amounts of protein on a daily basis. This requires some regular ingestion of at least small amounts of meat. A vegetarian certainly should take a balanced amino acid complex on a regular basis. Amino acids build protein and act as neu-rotransmitters or precursors of neu-rotransmitters (the chemicals that carry information from one nerve cell to another, providing energy directly to muscle tissue). Amino acids can also help absorb other required nutrients. Try to avoid taking large, regular doses of single amino acids, since the eventual accumulated imbalances in the body can exert their own toxicity. If you do supplement amino acids, take a balanced, complete spectrum of them.

Unless your supplements upset your stomach, consider taking them 30-60 minutes before meals with water or juice. Absorption can be variable when you take them with different types of foods. Consider taking a digestive enzyme such as pa-paya tablets with your supplements. This will help in their ab-sorption and then will help with the food you subsequently eat. Papaya is very inexpensive and very good for helping digestion.

Macrominerals
Common Minerals Present in the Body in Large Amounts

1. **Calcium:** Vital for the proper function of all cells; also essential for proper bone formation and maintenance; supplement ation is not generally recommended, except to acutely support healing.

   Even in the presence of osteoporosis, calcium supplementation has strong counterbalancing Negatives, promoting most other degenerative diseases, including cancer and heart disease; try to eliminate toxins (especially of dental origin) instead. In fact, G.C. Curhan, et al. demonstrated that high supplemental calcium may increase the risk of symptomatic kidney stones, while high dietary calcium intake appears to decrease this risk. *Common Dietary Sources: sardines, clams, oysters, turnip greens, mustard greens, broccoli, peas, beans, fruits.*

(Note that pasteurized milk and milk products, 'fortified' with vitamin D deliver too much calcium to tissues other than the bones, promoting degenerative diseases.)

2. **Chloride:** Major cellular anion (negative ion), maintaining pH balance, activating enzymes, and essential to the formation of hydrochloric acid in the stomach; except for using sodium chloride (table salt) to taste, no specific supplementation is required. *Common Dietary Sources: table salt, seafood, meat, eggs, soy sauce.*

3. **Magnesium:** Vital for bone formation; bio-available magnesium supplementation can increase bone mass; essential for acti-vating many different enzymes; involved in protein synthesis and nerve impulse transmission; consider supplementing with 20-100 milligrams of a properly chelated form. Higher doses can be used temporarily to help mobilize excess accumulations of calcium in the body, as reflected in hair analysis. *Common Dietary Sources: nuts, peas, beans, cereal grains, corn, carrots, seafood, brown rice, parsley, spinach.*

4. **Phosphorus:** "Companion" mineral to calcium; activator of many different enzymes; generally should not be supplemented for the same reasons as calcium. *Common Dietary Sources: meat, poultry, fish, eggs, nuts, peas, beans, grains.*

5. **Potassium:** Important cellular electrolyte; integrally involved with calcium and sodium in proper cellular membrane function; consider supplementing when blood or hair levels are low, but only with proper follow-up of subsequent blood or hair levels, with a competent health care practitioner. *Common Dietary Sources: avocado, fruits, potato, beans, tomato, wheat bran, eggs.*

6. **Sodium:** Important cellular electrolyte, along with calcium and potassium; generally needs only to be supplemented as table salt to taste. *Common Dietary Sources: table salt, meat, seafood, vegetables.*

7. **Sulfur:** Important component of some amino acids; should only consider supplementation with organic forms such as MSM (Methyl-Sulfonyl-Methane). *Common Dietary Sources: high-protein foods, e.g., meat, poultry, fish, eggs, peas, nuts, beans.*

Microminerals

Common Minerals Present in the Body in
Small or Trace Amounts

1. **Boron:** Important in bone strength and structure; consider supplementing with 100-200 micrograms daily of a chelated form. *Common Dietary Sources: fruits, vegetables, peas, beans, nuts.*

2. **Chromium:** Important in the proper interaction of insulin and blood glucose; consider supplementing with 25-50 micrograms daily of a chelated form. *Common Dietary Sources: prunes, nuts, asparagus, organ meats, grains.*

3. **Copper:** Required for the proper use of iron by the body; consider supplementing with about one milligram daily of a chelated form. *Common Dietary Sources: liver, seafood – especially shellfish, grains, peas, beans, nuts, eggs, meats, poultry.*

4. **Iodine:** Required for thyroid hormone synthesis; consider supplementing with about 150 micrograms daily of a form such as potassium iodide. *Common Dietary Sources: iodized salt, seafood, eggs, beef liver, peanuts, spinach, pumpkin, broccoli.*

5. **Iron:** Required for the synthesis of red blood cells; generally, a male should never supplement iron, since it can easily accumulate to toxic levels in the absence of loss by bleeding; a menstruating female should consider supplementing under the guidance of her health care practitioner. *Common Dietary Sources: meat, especially organ meats such as liver, clams and oysters, peas, beans, nuts, seeds, green leafy vegetables, fruits, grains, beets.*

6. **Manganese:** Important in normal brain function and numerous enzyme systems; consider supplementing with two to four milligrams daily of a chelated form. Common Dietary Sources: wheat bran, peas, beans, nuts, lettuce, blueberries, pineapple, seafood, poultry, meat.

7. **Molybdenum:** Important in the metabolism of the building blocks of DNA and RNA; consider supplementing with 10-20 micrograms daily of a chelated form. *Common Dietary Sources: soybeans, lentils, buckwheat, oats, rice.*

8. **Selenium:** Protects cells against free radicals; also helps neutralize heavy metals such as mercury; consider supplementing with 10-20 micrograms daily of a chelated form. Men with higher levels of selenium appear to have a lower risk of prostate cancer than men with lower levels. *Common Dietary Sources: grains, meats, poultry, fish.*

9. **Zinc:** Important in energy metabolism and the function of many enzymatic systems; consider supplementing with five to fifteen milligrams of a chelated form. *Common Dietary*

Sources: oysters, wheat germ, beef liver, dark poultry meats, grains.

Beware of taking a large variety of different multi-component supplements, as you can easily exceed the recommended dosages of the macrominerals, the microminerals, and the vitamins, to be discussed next. Many preparations like to throw in a variety of other nutrients along with the "featured" nutrient. Do your arithmetic, and don't overdo it!

Vitamins

As noted earlier, vitamins are already in an organic form. This is not to say that all purified vitamins are in an optimally bio-available form, as they would be in foods. However, a purified vitamin will be much closer to a food form than most minerals as found in the earth's crust. Having noted this distinction, it is nevertheless important to also find vitamins in forms as close to food forms as possible.

Many vitamins can be overdosed relatively easily. The main reason for this is that vitamins, while vital to proper bodily function, are needed in only the tiniest of amounts, as a general rule. When dealing with supplementation of any kind, you simply cannot assume that if a little is good, more must be better. Always remember that EVERYTHING is toxic in a high enough dose. No exceptions. And this includes many things that you require for survival. Everything in the biological sciences needs balance, and too much of something good should be avoided just as diligently as too little of it.

The vitamins comprise a very diverse group of organic substances. Although they are generally not related at all in their chemical structures or physiological roles, they are divided into two broad categories, related to their mechanisms of absorption into the body: water-soluble vitamins and fat-soluble vitamins.

There are Four Fat-Soluble Vitamins

1. **Vitamin A:** known to be essential for vision, the immune system, and for functions associated with proper growth; also an antioxidant; probably best supplemented as beta-carotene, which converts to vitamin A and minimizes the possibility of over-dosage. H. Melhus, et al, have shown that too much vitamin A is associated with reduced bone mineral density and increased risk for hip fracture. Common Dietary Sources: beef liver, sweet potato, carrots, spinach, butter nut squash.

2. **Vitamin D:** Known to be essential for good skeletal growth and strong bones; only minimal sunlight exposure is necessary to meet the daily requirement; this vitamin is EASILY overdosed and can promote abnormal calcification throughout the body, as it increases calcium absorption from the gut; the increased calcium absorbed does not seek out the bones, how-ever. M.S. Schwartzman and W.A. Franck demonstrated that pharmacological doses of vitamin D will worsen osteoporosis; consider not supplementing this vitamin at all unless in close coordination with your health care provider, making sure that the desired clinical effects are being accomplished. Common Dietary Sources: few natural dietary sources; present in fortified milk (not recommended, see above).

3. **Vitamin E:** Known to help maintain the integrity of cellular membranes in the body; also an antioxidant; try to take preparations with as much "d-alpha-tocopherol" content as possible; generally do not exceed 800 IU per day; a chronic dosage of 400 IU daily would probably be advisable for most. Common Dietary Sources: vegetable seed oils, peanuts. Lesser amounts in many different fresh vegetables and fruits.

4. **Vitamin K:** Necessary for proper blood clotting; does not generally need supplementation unless some form of malabsorption exists in the gut, or if the bacteria in the gut that manufactures this vitamin have been destroyed. *Common Dietary Sources: green leafy vegetables, soybeans, beef liver.*

J. M. Rapola, et. al. recently published in the *Lancet* that beta-carotene significantly increased the number of fatal heart attacks among men with previous heart attack who smoked. Without a good explanation of why this effect has been observed, it would be safest to advise smoking men who have known heart disease to avoid beta-carotene and other vitamin A supplementation completely for the time being. However, an epidemiological study suggests that a diet rich in beta-carotene might lower a woman's risk of breast cancer after menopause, so a complete avoidance of beta-carotene supplementation is not being recommended at this time. Further research may be needed to determine if supplemented beta-carotene is less desirable than dietary beta-carotene. Certainly, as a general rule, supplemented nutrients can never be as desirable as dietary nutrients.

The fat-soluble vitamins noted above are absorbed along with dietary fats. Normally, these vitamins are not excreted into the urine, tending to be stored in the body in moderate amounts. Conversely, the water-soluble vitamins are more numerous, are excreted in the urine, and are not stored in the body in appre-ciable quantities. Some lists may include additional compounds considered by some to fit the definition of a vitamin. Here is a list of water-soluble vitamins considered by most authorities to be complete:

Water-Soluble Vitamins

1. **Vitamin B1** (thiamin): Known to be essential in helping to generate cellular energy, to promote fatty acid synthesis, and to support normal membrane and nerve conduction; little

toxicity has been observed with high oral intakes; unless a deficiency exists, consider supplementing with a dose ranging from 5-25 mg daily. *Common Dietary Sources: yeast, sunflower seeds, peas, beans.*

2. **Vitamin B2** (riboflavin): Important in the cellular reactions that transfer energy from one chemical substance to another; also serves as an antioxidant; helps in the formation of energy from food fats and proteins; deficiency syndrome has not been clearly characterized; consider supplementing with a dose ranging from 5-15mg daily. *Common Dietary Sources: beef liver, meat, oysters.*

3. **Vitamin B3** (niacin): Important for the proper function of numerous enzymes; important in the synthesis of multiple hormones; important for proper function of the brain and nervous system; deficiency results in a syndrome called pellagra; 5-20 mg daily dosage probably acceptable for most people; niacin can excessively accelerate detoxification in susceptible individuals, common in those who have their dental toxicity removed. *Common Dietary Sources: beef and beef liver, poultry, fish.*

4. **Vitamin B6** (commonly, pyridoxine): Important for the proper function of multiple enzymes involved in amino acid metabolism; consider supplementing with a dose ranging from 5-15 mg daily. *Common Dietary Sources: meat, beans, potato, banana.*

5. **Folic acid:** Important in the synthesis of DNA and the metabolism of amino acids and histidine; consider supplementing with 200-400 micrograms daily. *Common Dietary Sources: brewer's yeast, spinach, asparagus, turnip greens, lima beans, beef liver.*

6. **Vitamin C** (ascorbic acid): Felt to be important in numerous aspects of physiology, including fat metabolism, immune function and healing, endocrine function, and neutralization of toxicity; also an antioxidant; important to take adequate doses on a regular basis; many individuals will do best on 10-15 grams of sodium ascorbate daily, taken under the direction of their health care provider. *Common Dietary Sources: papaya, orange, cantaloupe, broccoli, brussel sprouts, green peppers, grapefruit, strawberries.*

7. **Vitamin B12** (cobalamins): Important for the maintenance of proper nerve function and blood synthesis; unless a clear defi-ciency syndrome exists (pernicious anemia and/or markedly low blood levels of the vitamin), consider avoiding any supplemen-tation with this vitamin, as supplement forms of B12 can promote the methylation of inorganic mercury in the body, making it much more toxic and causing clinical compromise. *Common Dietary Sources: meat, seafood, poultry.*

8. **Biotin:** Important in the energy metabolism of the body; consider supplementing with 100-200 micrograms daily. *Common Dietary Sources: yeast, liver, kidney.*

9. **Pantothenic acid:** A precursor to the body's synthesis of its own coenzyme A; important in the metabolism of carbohydrates and fats; consider supplementing with 10-20 mg daily. *Common Dietary Sources: widespread, especially high in egg yolk, liver, kidney, yeast.*

Eating Habits for suggested periods of therapy: Cut down on fatty foods. Substitute red meat with fish, or fowl, vegetables, whole grains, nuts, fruits, and healthy juices. Make sure your protein intake is adequate.

The preceding text on 'Vitamins and Minerals, by Dr. Thomas Levy, is published here with his permission. Please see Appendix A on Hair Analysis, to determine vitamin/mineral overload and/or deficiency.

Diet and Nutrition

"Let food be your medicine and medicine your food."
Hippocrates

Most of us know the importance of healthy eating. We hear about it every other day. It comes to us in some form or another as a nagging reminder from our doctors, television commentators, concerned family members and well-meaning friends. Most moms, of course, offer us their best kitchen remedies when it comes to our health.

Eating is more than just fuel for the fire. It turns out that "food" can be our best friend or our worst enemy. Four of the leading causes of death in the United States are linked to food while, on the other hand, food has been listed as a contributing factor in curing such ailments as acne, constipation, arthritis, and high cholesterol. The list goes on.

Modern pharmaceuticals treat the symptoms of our ailments, and while they often work, we should regard the symptoms as a warning sign. Although a drug might alleviate the symptom, it does not treat the cause. Our body is signaling that something needs to be changed, usually in the way of diet, cleanliness, stress or environment. Ignore the cause, and even the drugs we rely on can lead to disease.

It's beneficial to take control of our own health and while the primary focus of this book is biomagnetics, we would like to touch briefly on the subject of nutrition and how proper diet can enhance the healing process.

BODY BASICS

To better understand how nutrition affects the living system, it is important to discuss the basic structure and function of our body. The cell is the basic structural and functional component of life. It is composed of two or more atoms linked together called molecules. The overall function of the cell is to obtain energy from organic nutrients, synthesize complex molecules such as protein, eliminate waste and duplicate itself. In the human body there are over 200 distinct types of cells, which are broken down into four basic classifications:

Epithelial cells form boundaries between compartments, act as selective barriers and regulate the secretion and absorption of ions and organic molecules across the membrane. Muscle cells are responsible for locomotion, movement of materials through the body, and contractual ability in response to stimuli.

Connective-tissue cells are the connecting, anchoring, and supporting structures. Blood, bone, fat, and cartilage are examples of different connective tissues.

Nerve cells initiate and conduct electrical impulses. These cells, when grouped together with similar cells that perform specific functions are called organs. Although their job is complex, when working properly, they create an internal environment where the cells can survive and function.

This internal environment is named extracellular fluid. Most of this fluid, called interstitial fluid, surrounds the cells while the remainder is the fluid portion of blood, commonly known as blood plasma. Our internal environment must maintain the correct chemical balance in order for us to survive.

Water, oxygen, food, vitamins, and minerals play an important role in maintaining this process. For example, food nutrients are broken down into small molecules by the digestive system. These molecules move from the lumen of the gastrointestinal tract and are absorbed into the blood plasma. They are then distributed throughout the body by the circulatory systems to interstitial fluid surrounding the cells. A complex exchange mechanism occurs. Carbon dioxide, waste and other metabolic products pass out of the cell while oxygenated nutrients, minerals, vitamins and water go in.

The cell membrane, made up of lipids and proteins, controls the passage of these nutrients by way of diffusion, mediated transport, osmosis or endo/exocytosis.

Proteins in the cell membrane provide pathways for selective entrance of nutrients and minerals, while the lipid layer prevents the movement of molecules through the membrane, partly because the extremities of the lipid bilayer are nonpolar (no charge). Ions, such as NA+ (sodium) or K+ (potassium) have to diffuse through protein channels. This is accomplished by the electric charge difference across the plasma membrane. Remember that most cells have a net Negative charge inside the cell that attracts Positive ions in and Negative ions out.

When all organs function properly, the cell maintains a working chemical balance between intracellular metabolism and the internal environment for optimum health. This is called homeostasis.

The body, of course, has a defense mechanism to main-tain homeostasis, but this doesn't mean that the cell can say to a toxic nitrate, "I do not select you. You're toxic." In other words, foreign chemicals such as nitrates found in processed foods are also metabolized. The body absorbs and stores these toxins as readily as it does good nutrients. Major storage sites are bone, fat and cell proteins.

Bone marrow produces erythrocytes (new red blood cells) The life-span of an erythrocyte is about 120 days. That means that our body is replacing old red blood cells at a rate of about 100 billion cells daily. Blood carries oxygen and nutrients to every cell, and is necessary for cellular metabolism. Protein is the major building block of every cell. It is the main ingredient of DNA, our genetic and cellular toolbar, and it plays an important structural role in the makeup of the cellular membrane. Fat acts as a major insulator, a source of energy and is also a structural part of the cell membrane.

A build up of toxins or foreign chemicals, to any or all of these three important tissues can add stress to the little hard-working cells that work even harder when trying to maneuver around toxic build-ups. Storage in the way of 'too much of a good thing' leads to high cholesterol, high blood pressure, or toxic accumulation and can damage the cell's structure and function. Just a simple blockage in our body's electrochemical pathway can cause a 'short circuit' in any one of our body's systems.

What we put into our body should provide the cell with nourishment, and while the body can metabolize and excrete many foreign chemicals, these foreign invaders are best avoided. In fact, most of us understand we need to eat foods from the basic food groups in amounts that don't lead to accumulation.

Why does our body need certain nutrients and minerals? The answer is in our body composition. Our body is made up of hydrogen (H), oxygen (0), carbon (C), and nitrogen (N), atoms which account for 99.3% of the essential elements, while minerals and trace elements make up the remaining essential chemical elements. These three elements, (H, 0, and N) together with carbon, form the major categories of organic molecules that exist in the body.

Carbohydrates (C,H2O). About 1% of our body weight; carbohydrate literally means water-containing carbon atoms, and plays an important role in cellular energy production. Sugars such as monosaccharides and disaccharides are a subclass of carbohydrates. Carbohydrates are broken down in the intestine by digestive enzymes and converted into sugars such as glucose, which are then stored as glycogen or fat or used for energy.

Lipids (C,H). Approximately 15% of our body weight. Triglycerols (fats), phospholipids (lipid linked to a phosphate), steroids (cholesterol, cortisol, estrogen, testosterone) are subclasses. Fatty acids + glycerol are subunits. The body makes most of the fat it needs. Lipids are insoluble in water and play an important role as electrical insulators, energy supply and structural components of the cell membrane.

Proteins (C,H2O,N). Approximately 17% of our body weight. The subclasses are peptides, and proteins. The subunits are amino acids. Protein plays a critical part in cell structure and cell metabolism. Enzymes, hormones and antibodies are also made up of proteins.

Nucleic acids (C,H2O,N). About 2% body weight. Subclasses are DNA and RNA. Subunits are Nucleotides. Stores and transmits genetic information.

Carbohydrates, Protein, Amino Acids, and Fats. Most of us recognize these words. Besides being words associated with diet, one can see, they are different combinations of the essential elements that make up our body composition.

Certain nutrients are essential to sustain life. They are nutrients that must be supplied by our diet because they cannot be synthesized in adequate amounts by our body and they are essential to life.

Essential Nutrients. Water is the number one essential nutrient comprising 60% of our body mass. Besides water, there are 9 essential amino acids, 7 major minerals, 13 trace minerals, 2 essential fatty acids – linoleic and linolenic, water and fat soluble vitamins and a few other essential ingredients.

It doesn't mean we have to eat meat to get protein, nor does it mean there are only 7 major minerals that our body needs. These are the norm; definitions that have been generally accepted.

For instance, there are 22 amino acids that make up a protein. The body can synthesize all but 9 of these, which it must get from our diet. Many foods when combined, such as beans and corn, with the right vegetable, will make up a complete protein.

Some regular intake of meat and animal food is important unless it infringes on your beliefs. In that case, it is important to make sure you are getting adequate protein beans, nuts, etc.

The list of essential nutrients may change over time with the discovery of new information. So it is important for anyone serious about his/her health, to purchase a good book on nutrition and keep abreast of current information. Our body needs these nutrients to maintain the chemical balance between the cell and the internal environment. An overload of the wrong chemicals, such as those found in processed foods, or a shortage of the right nutrients will cause a chemical imbalance. Because the body function is so complex, the pain in your gut could be the chemical result of what you initially put in your mouth.

While proper cellular metabolism is dependent upon nutrients, minerals, oxygen and water to maintain health, there is still no definitive answer to the age-old quest for the eternal fountain of youth. Although the right nutrition won't help you live forever, it will add quality for a more healthful life.

As Hippocrates said, "The life so short,
the craft so long to learn."

Summary of Diet and Nutrition

Biomagnetism can help reorganize and balance the electrical nature of the cells for advanced healing. However, it is absolutely essential that cells have the right building blocks (water, oxygen, vitamins, minerals and food nutrients) to maintain the cure. Often, illness comes from a vitamin/mineral/food deficiency. Cure the deficiency and the illness will disappear.

CHAPTER TEN

Harmful Effects Of Electricity And High Voltage Power Lines

Did you know that in Sweden it is illegal to have a workspace where an employee is subjected to an EMF (electromagnetic field) from Alternating Current that is over 2mG (two milligauss – two-thousandths of one gauss)? Why? Because Swedish governmental scientific tests have shown that human tissue, subjected to this type of field for extended periods of time, has a reasonable probability of developing cancer.

What is EMF?

A basic law of physics is that magnetic fields stimulate (excite) electrons – that is how electricity is made. Electricity is generated by passing wires through multiple magnetic fields (60 per second here in the USA and 50ps on most other continents). This pulses and stimulates the electrons, making them flow through the wires to be used as electricity elsewhere. Without magnetic fields, there would be no electricity, which means no lights, appliances, electronic devices, transportation, flight, or any contemporary technology as we know it.

Another law of physics: Everything that transmits and uses electricity gives off EMF (Electromagnetic Fields). High tension wires transmit EMF up to 100 yards during the summer air conditioning season. Appliances such as cordless phones, stoves, stereos and electronic devices like laptops or tablets transmit fairly powerful, pulsing EMF short distances, while Wifi and cell phones transmit lower-powered EMF long distances. This means that strong and weak EMFs are constantly going through our body – but what does that mean to our health?

Our body is made up of billions of atoms in complex arrangements called molecules that form our cells and tissue. All atoms have electrons that naturally spin around their nucleus which, consolidated in a cell, give off voltage readings. Since 1939, it has been established by the medical community and recognized by the US FDA that [bio-cellular] electrical analysis of cellular voltage gives an instant and precise "snapshot" diagnosis of how healthy cells are and how well they are functioning (metabolizing).

In other words, the cell's voltage is simply an electrical measurement of its health. Cells that measure in the higher voltage range [of electromotive vitality] are healthy and in homeostasis with good immune function. Cells that measure in the low voltage range are dysfunctioning and indicative of people with poor immune functions who are ill with symptoms like chronic fatigue syndrome, fibromyalgia and/or many other chronic medical conditions.

How does EMF affect our health?

The electrons of a cell and its metabolic functions are directly affected by EMF. Electricity is made from pulsed magnetic fields that energize the electrons, and so the pulsing EMF emitted from appliances and electronic devices directly affects the electrons in our cells. As the EMF pervades the cells, the electrons' natural free spin is altered and disrupted by the pulsing fields. Over a period of time, the external EMF can disrupt the electron spin enough to wear down the cell's voltage, leading to cellular dysfunction, poor health, and altered DNA.

Worldwide research shows that EMF as small as over 2mG (milligauss), over a period of time, can disrupt and lower the cell's voltage and functionality; subsequently the body may gov into chronic fatigue syndrome, malabsorption, Parkinson's, MS, cancer, etc.

Daily, we are dosed with EMF from cordless phones (15mG), Ipads (20mG), laptop computers (25-50mG), dashboards of cars (50mG) and many other electrical devices such as the new powerfully transmitting Electric Smart Meters. We live in an environment of constant EMF attack.

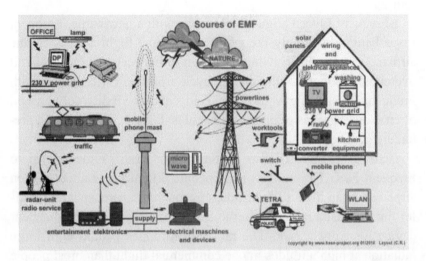

Years ago when alarm clock plug-in radios came out, there was a large increase of brain tumors from the strong EMF to the head from sleeping within one meter of the radio. Now EMF is everywhere and everyone should consider some form of protection.

Jet Lag and Frequent Flyer Fatigue

Jet Lag is a perfect example of a symptom of a major EMF attack. The EMF in the interior of a commercial airplane has been measured at over 100mG. The airplane interior is really a big milligauss oven where everyone is baked by EMF for the entire flight. Many people are quite aware of their jet lag, yet have no idea that EMF plays a large role in their reaction.

A healthy researcher who worked with us abhorred flying because it would disorient her for almost a week after a flight. A woman flight attendant in her mid-forties with many years on the job came in for a consultation and explained how she and her colleagues were always sick and tired with colds and headaches. She also told us that a fairly large percentage of the retired flying community, instead of enjoying their golden years, got ill and died within a few years of retiring.

Frequent Flyer Fatigue is old news with a new name. Frequent Flyer Fatigue is simply the result of multiple flight attacks by the airplane's strong EMF without enough in-between time to heal and overcome the low cellular energy cycle from the EMF. People with Frequent Flyer Fatigue have lowered cellular vitality/voltage and often show the signs of poor health, colds, fatigue, insomnia and pre-mature aging.

However, there is also another major health issue related to Frequent Flyer Fatigue that most people do not know about. When airplanes fly in high altitudes, there is much less atmosphere to buf-fer the increased radiation in the cabin from the big thermonuclear device we call the sun. The radiation saturates people with more radiation at high altitudes in one commercial flight than most people receive who work full time in the nuclear power industry.

BiomagScience suggests using Biomagnetic therapy in conjunc-tion with vitamin C daily to provide the minimum anti-oxidant "donor electrons" to supplement the body with enough healing energy to overcome the massive amount of free-radicals from the radiation.

The Best EMF Protection for Your Body
Is High Cellular Vitality/Voltage

EMF is not able to electrically degrade the cells of someone who is healthy and has a high electromotive cellular vitality/voltage. A large EMF attack like that from a commercial flight may wear them down a little for a short time, but their high cellular vitality returns rapidly and their health bounces back immediately.

However, for individuals who have had their energy (voltage) continuously robbed and degraded by EMF from using cordless and cell phones, sitting or sleeping too close to a stereo or plug-in radio, using a laptop all the time on their lap, or perhaps sleeping against the wall that backs up to their refrigerator, they can develop an unfortunate downward spiral of poor health that can lead to illness and premature death. This is evident from the massive amount of EMF research from all over the world.

Gadgets to Counter and Protect from EMF

There are numerous types and shapes of pendants, crystals, earthing pads and electronic devices that promise to absorb, neutralize, harmonize, and energize the pulsed EMF to protect the body. Although the earthing pad can be very good, it also can pick up stray current feedback or what is called dirty electricity – this is something you should check before using it. Most of the gadgets have a small effect on people. But none of them has the electromotive power to measurably and immediately increase the cellular voltage and health that BiomagScience energy supplementation does by simply wearing a magnet.

The Best Defense from EMF – Keep Your Cells Charged

When BiomagScience consulted with the above-mentioned flight attendant, her voltage measurements were so low it was apparent her cells were dysfunctional and her immune system was compromised; that is why she was constantly tired with a cold and a headache. After an hour of energizing her body with Daytime Therapy, her cellular voltage bumped up and she said she 'suddenly did not feel tired.' Then over the next month, she reported her cold, headache and fatigue went away and that she 'had not felt so good in so many years, she had forgotten the earlier feeling.' She was so excited she wanted to establish a BiomagScience clinic in Chile where she lived.

The researcher, who hated to fly because of the long-term disorientation from jet lag, finally took a flight while she was using the

Daytime therapy. After landing, she couldn't believe there was no disorientation; the same with her return trip – no disorientation at all. The Daytime Therapy protected her from the EMF attack.

We were not surprised that the researcher did not experience her unusual jet lag, because after so many years of research and applied magnetic therapy, these results were common even in the most unusual cases. However, with the Bio-cellular Analysis technology, we were finally able to measure and evaluate how our therapies increased electromotive vitality, which gave us a greater understanding in developing more advanced therapies. See "cellular before and after voltage tests" under "Research" at www.BiomagScience.Net.

There was a case of a man who developed bad health after taking a new job. This was unusual since this individual had been very healthy all his life. Since starting the new job, every winter he experienced an allergic type respiratory condition which led to sleeping problems, colds and an overall lack of vitality. His doctor prescribed antibiotics, antihistamines and sleeping pills, but nothing seemed to work.

At a later time, he moved to another office and his health immediately returned. We examined his former office and found a large electric heater and fan motor on the ceiling just under the floor where he sat at his desk. Each day that he sat at his desk during the wintertime, he was being bombarded with very strong EMF. Fortunately for him, his health rebounded when he moved away from the EMF field.

BiomagScience worked with an individual who was so electrically sensitive to EMF, she couldn't be in the house when the refrigerator or the air conditioning fan was running. She finally escaped to a cabin in the mountains with no electricity. At the time, we didn't measure cellular voltage, but we are certain that her voltage readings were extremely low. We started her slowly on Biomagnetic therapy baby steps and over a period of time, she was able to build up her energy/ voltage and resume a normal life.

Every sick or chronically ill person we measured had low cellular voltage readings before magnetic therapy and substantially higher readings after therapy. Numerous times, the voltage would go up more in an hour of therapy than six months of a specialized diet could provide nutritionally. As the voltage went up, each individual's health got better.

A healthy body is the best protection from EMF

The first step to protect yourself is, using the One-Meter Rule, move all your plug-in clocks, stereos, older tube computer screens, older TV tube screens, or anything electronic that plugs in one meter (39.6 inches) or further away from where you sit or sleep or work. Then that type of EMF field will not invade your space. You might want to get an inexpensive milligauss meter to check your home and work. They are available in hardware stores. See cell phone below.

Smart Meters have a far-reaching field which has been shown to give young children leukemia and poor health, and to cause tumors and cancer in adults. All the information is on the Web. To protect yourself, go online and get an EMF safety cover to stop the bad EMF from invading your house. To protect yourself from your neighbor's too-close Smart Meter, tell him about it and make sure he gets one too.

Maintaining High Cellular Vitality is the Best EMF Defense

Since people with high cellular voltage/vitality are not affected by EMF, then maintaining that vitality is a must and simple to do. This is easily achieved with BiomagScience's Daytime therapy and drinking 2-4 glasses of Bio-Negative Energized Water, which further helps increase vitality through hydration and cellular nutrition and detoxification. Used daily, this simple, healthy energetic supplementation helps maintain high cellular vitality/voltage and helps prevent disease from EMF.

Daily energy supplementation is also a must for cell phone users. It will help prevent tumors and long term disorientation from EMF output.

Note: When you are flying, BioMagnets normally do not set off the airport metal detector, but it is advised to wear the BioMagnets under your clothing so you do not have to go through the process of explaining what you health magnets are.

Here are two very thorough books on this subject:

WARNING: The Electricity Around You May Be Hazardous to Your Health, by Ellen Sugarman, published by Simon and Schuster.

The Great Power-Line Cover-Up by Paul Brodeur, published by Back Bay Books, Little Brown and Company.

CHAPTER ELEVEN

DENTAL TOXICITY
By Tom Levy

BiomagScience wants you to be aware of one of the main causes of poor health. This chapter was developed by leading practitioners worldwide who are knowledgeable about dental toxity, one of the worst health problems in our society, and what can be done to prevent it.

Toxicity from any source will detract from good health. Substantial data exists to indicate that dental toxicity represents a dominant source of toxicity in most of the citizens of developed nations today. Therefore, a greater awareness of this toxicity and how to minimize its presence and impact are vitally important to any seeker of optimum health.

Overview

Toxicity from any source can operate by at least one of two mechanisms:

1. Toxins can directly bind to and damage different tissues and enzyme systems in the body.

2. Toxins can damage and impair the ability of the immune system to protect the body from any insult. This includes further damage from other toxins.

Toxins can contribute to poor health in other ways, but these two mechanisms are among the most important to consider and understand.

Mercury and Heavy Metals

The most common type of dental fillings routinely used for over the past one hundred years are amalgam fillings. Also commonly known as silver fillings, these materials are actually comprised of approximately 50% mercury when first placed! Mercury is the most toxic, non-radioactive heavy metal known to man. To make things worse, mercury in its un-combined state as well as in its amalgamated state continually produces mercury vapor. This vapor can be directly inhaled inside the mouth, or it can be rapidly converted to organic forms or inorganic salts in the mouth and after swallowing. It has already been conclusively shown that the more mercury amalgams you have in your mouth, the more mercury you have in your brain. A mere five such fillings can increase brain mercury levels threefold.

Mercury is toxic to everybody, requiring no special sensitivity. However, some people can be more sensitive than others and can have additional negative health effects beyond the direct toxic effects of the mercury. This does not mean that anyone who does not demonstrate any of the relatively rare "allergic" reactions to mercury will still not suffer the generalized toxic effects from exposure to it.

Although the mercury in the filling is the most toxic component, the rest of the components include tin, silver, copper and zinc from elemental sources. Such forms of these metals are also highly toxic to most people. Metals in your mouth are not only chemically toxic, but can also generate small electrical currents, causing another form of dental toxicity.

Electrical Dental Toxicity

The phenomenon is called oral galvanism. By using a probe and a micro ammeter, these tiny currents can be easily measured. The measurements consistently recorded from amalgams, crowns, braces, and other metals in the mouth, range from 1-100 microamperes and sometimes even higher. Further, the polarity of the current can be in a Positive or Negative orientation. Clinically, high Positive voltage readings seem to correlate with the sickest patients.

The electricity in the mouth can impact the patient in at least two significant ways. The highest current readings in a given mouth can be as much as 5,000 to 7,000 times greater than the currents measured in the normally functioning brain. The natural currents found in the brain run only in the range of seven to nine nanoamperes (a billionth of an ampere). A "hot" reading in the upper jawbone allows a huge chronic electrical current to reside only about an inch away from the exquisitely sensitive brain and central nervous system. It's not hard to see how such a current could completely overwhelm the ability of a nearby area of the brain to sense its own much tinier currents. In fact, a number of patients with uncontrollable seizure activity showed immediate and dramatic improvements when amalgam fillings were removed.

The electrical activity of metals in the mouth also affects the rate of release of mercury from amalgam fillings. The greater the electromotive difference (potential) between amalgam and another metal in the mouth, the greater the "pressure" available to push out mercury vapor. This tends to be especially pronounced when gold is placed in a mouth with amalgam. Gold by itself is a good dental metal for most people. However, when gold is near amalgam, as is the case with a gold crown on top of an old amalgam filling, mercury vapor release will escalate. Clinical deterioration is often seen when new gold crowns are placed on top of old amalgam fillings.

Truth be known, there are so many different forms of dental toxicity that it would be very difficult to ever say that any one component is the primary problem for a given symptom. In addition to the difficulty in figuring out what is causing what, low-dose mercury poisoning has long been an elusive diagnosis that is rarely made. Individuals poisoned with mercury are often written off as hypochondriacs, due largely to the subtlety of the symptoms. Among the symptoms that can be manifest are included irritability, depression, insomnia, nervousness, mild tremor, impaired judgment and coordination, decreased clarity and efficiency of thought, emotional instability, ADD, MS, headache, fatigue, and loss of sex drive. If it seems that everyone has one or more of these symptoms, it is no coincidence, since nearly the entire population has amalgam fillings.

What Can Be Done To Help Combat Dental Toxicity?

Replacement dental materials can be costly and also cause a lot of harm to ones health. In fact, certain chemicals in some replacement fillings can be just as clinically damaging as the amalgam. If you become motivated to get your dental fillings changed, choose a dentist who is informed about dental toxicity and consider using blood bio-compatibility testing to give you the best possible chance at finding replacement materials that do not further damage your immune system.

Biomagnetic therapy can be very effective in stimulating the immune system to fight whatever toxicity is present, alleviating some of the symptoms. It has been shown that a very toxic person can be made clinically well by the proper usage of magnets.

BioMagnetic Therapy for Dental Toxicity

Place the Negative 2-Stack Power Wafers on the back of the neck. The proper Negative field will energize all of the cells in the tissue between the amalgams and the nervous system near the brain stem. The vitalized cells will now create an obstacle that stops the deteriorating effects of the electrical currents emanating from the amalgams. In addition, as indicated in the chapter "Playing with Fire," the entire body will be energized, which increases immune system functions.

Biomagnetic therapy has been shown to help relieve symptoms due to dental toxicity. Proper use of medically calibrated magnets can be an excellent method of complementary therapy for anyone suffering from dental toxicity. However, symptoms could persist as the continuous release of mercury toxins has a harmful effect that works against the immune system. If this is the case, consult with a holistic dentist who is open and informed about toxins created by mercury and other heavy metals used in dentistry. Consider replacing the amalgams with an alternative substance that does not cause an allergic reaction to your body.

Using the ATACC (Acute Chronic Therapy Protocols) in the *Wellness Pictorial Guide* or in this book, Organ Group Energizing Therapy, Meridian Energizing Therapy, Daytime, Nightime, Bio-Negative Water, BAO and good nutrition has been shown to give a fairly rapid return to health after amalgam issues are eliminated.

Regaining lost health can be a difficult process, requiring a new lifestyle and much attention to detail. Removing toxicity or minimizing toxicity from as many sources as possible is one of the most important things to be done in this quest for better health. Using Biomagnetism can help regain health.

For further information on dental toxicity, dentists who specialize in dental toxicity, and blood biocompatibility testing, see Appendix A, "Peak Energy Performance."

Summary

Toxins can directly bind to and damage tissues in the body, impairing the ability of the immune system to protect the body from insult. Mercury and other heavy metals in the mouth can be both chemically and electrically toxic. Root canals, cavitations, dental implants and extractions for dentures can also introduce bacteria that metabolize oxygen from the mouth into an oxygen-starved environment. Oxygen-requiring bacteria, deprived of oxygen, produce toxic by-products resulting in toxicity levels much greater than botulism in some human enzyme systems.

Use BiomagScience therapies to alleviate toxic dental symptoms. Do what you can to improve your health and eliminate whatever bothersome symptoms you may have. Don't neglect being thorough in eliminating as many toxic assaults as possible from your body and your immune system. Pay special attention: remove as much of your dental toxicity as possible to help reach your best long-term health.

To treat dental toxicity, see "Toxicity in Health Problems and Therapies," Chapter 19.

CHAPTER TWELVE

HOW BIOMAGNETISM HELPS RELIEVE THE
PAIN FROM ARTHRITIS AND INFLAMMATION

The Earth and every element and living thing have magnetic fields. BiomagScience is the science of how to use specifically designed magnetic fields to increase the electrical charge of the human cells from their stressed, low energy, traumatized state back to their normal healthy state.

Arthritis pain comes from cellular inflammation of the tissue. And often arthritis occurs when MDS (magnetic deficiency syndrome, low cellular voltage) creates metabolic dysfunction and waste buildup in the cells by reducing their ability to transfer nutrition and oxygen and detoxify normally. Arthritic inflammation usually manifests itself in the extremities such as the hands, feet, wrists, ankles, then knees, elbows, etc. and affects circulation, cell and nerve function of joints, connective tissue, and muscles.

Connective tissue is found throughout the entire body. In a joint, the health of connective tissue is directly related to synovial or joint fluid. When there is a lowering of cellular voltage (MDS – Magnetic Deficiency Syndrome), bone tissue at the joints can be a prime storage area for toxins such as lead, mercury, arsenic and nitrates because the lowered energy value prohibits the exchange of nutrients and detoxification. This leads to a buildup of toxins which creates inflammation (arthritis) and further degeneration of the joint.

Arthritic inflammation also leads to improper targeting of calcium which painfully builds up in the joints and connective tissue, creating more inflammation and inhibiting healing. Cellular inflammation is like free radicals inasmuch as it always measures a Positive charge versus the normal Negative charge of healthy cells.

Biomagnetism Used Successfully to Treat Arthritis

Biomagnetism is a safe, non-invasive therapy to help overcome the crippling effects of arthritis. The biomagnet provides the healing Bio-Negative energy that charges the cells, helping overcome the MDS. This in turn normalizes the cellular dysfunction that is causing the inflammation. The biomagnet emits the Bio-Negative charge, which penetrates through the skin to stimulate and increase the dysfunctional cell's low voltage so that it has the ability to dispel the accumulated waste products out of the cell into the circulatory system for elimination.

The process of overcoming the MDS with Biomagnetism that helps normalize the cells provides fairly rapid pain relief as the inflammation is eliminated and circulation is increased. This provides oxygen, water, electrolytes, proteins, hemoglobin, hormones and other nutrients needed to support healthy cells and homeostasis. After the first pain relief, the therapy should be carried on for another two weeks to ensure the site heals.

Another important part of the therapy is to systemically charge the entire body with the Daytime and Nightime therapies, along with Bio-Negative water with BAO (BiomagScience Activated Oxygen) and adequate nutrition. These protocols will help the entire body overcome the MDS that is causing the arthritis.

Biomagnets Can Help Nerve Communication

As shown in regeneration of severed nerves, the biomagnetic energy stimulates nerve cells and their activity at the therapy site. Nerve cells send and receive electrical signals, and when working normally, transmit the required neuro-messages throughout the body to keep it healthy.

For example, when a trauma occurs such as hurting your leg, the area will go into a Positive charge state which will send an [ascending] message/signal to the brain, which will compute and send back the [descending] signal to flood the area with healing Bio-Negative energy. MDS (Magnetic Deficiency Syndrome) or trauma affects the nerve cells by reducing their electrical current which reduces the neuro-messaging communication the body is dependent upon for healing and homeostasis. The communication of the nervous system also plays an important role in stimulating the chemical messengers known as neurotransmitters. Neurotransmitters have many functions including nourishing the cells; telling the body there is pain; releasing endorphins, a natural analgesic or pain reliever; and sending natural Bio-Negative energy to flood the site to neutralize the Positive charged inflammation, thus healing the site.

When the nerve cells and their signals are weakened by stress or MDS and cannot communicate normally, the Bio-Negative energy applied over the inflamed site also charges the nerve cells to help them communicate normally for supportive healing.

Magnetized Energized Water and Arthritis

The buildup of waste products in tissue can lead to many health problems ranging from general fatigue to cancer. Water plays one of the most important roles in elimination of waste products and toxins from the body. Without sufficient water, dehydration causes the extracellular fluid to lose electrical conductivity. Without that conductivity, the cells lose the ability to metabolize.

Bio-Negatively energized structured water breaks up the grape-like molecular clusters (associations) into much smaller single and micronized clusters that can pass more easily into and out of the cells. While making the oxygen and hydrogen ions more accessible for cellular metabolism, the glands and organs, the smaller energized water components deliver more nutrients, oxygen and energy into the cells and carry more toxins out of the cells, supporting increased functionality and better cellular health.

Summary

Drinking great-tasting Bio-Negative water along with the Daytime therapy enhances the communication network within the neural, endocrine, genetic and circulatory systems, resulting in an improved immune system which can overcome arthritis. Our body needs proper nutrients and water to heal and BioMagnetics helps provide efficient delivery and increased metabolic functionality of these essential requirements along with the amplifying of the body's own healing energy, helping to return us to health and wellness.

BiomagScience research indicates there is a strong link between MDS (Magnetic Deficiency Syndrome) and the pain of arthritis or inflammation, and the pain can be reduced and often resolved by elevating the cellular vitality and overcoming the MDS.

CHAPTER THIRTEEN

BIOMAGNIFICENT TESTIMONIALS & CASE STUDIES

The art of helping the body heal itself with biomagnets has influenced many people. The following testimonials are written either in first person or taken from case studies.

My Ailing Heart

Mr. Alfred Ayers suffered in pain and discomfort. He couldn't walk more than 100 meters without gasping for breath, and then only aided with his cane. His doctor diagnosed his problem as coronary thrombosis and told him without bypass surgery, he wouldn't live more than 5 years.

Mr. Ayers had neither the money, nor insurance to cover the operation. He was extremely worried and anxious when a close friend encouraged him to wear this "new gadget" called a BioMagnet as a pendant. That was 1994. In April of 1995, Mr. Ayers returned to his doctor for a checkup. He was not surprised to find out that his heart condition had healed without surgery or expensive medicines because he could walk long distances now, and climb overpasses with ease and without his cane.

Mr. Ayers states, "At present, I still wear my BioMags for maintenance... Perhaps it's worth mentioning here that as a bonus, Biomags helped me get rid of my arthritis. Thank you BioMags."
~ Mr. Ayers

Seizures Eliminated

In yet another case study, a doctor by profession and mother of a nine-year-old boy shares the following testimonial:

"It's no joke playing mother to an adopted nine-year-old boy who is an epileptic. Imagine seeing him suffer grand mal seizures despite unpleasant medications such as Tegretol 200 mg. that he had to take three times daily. But things changed for the better when one day, I brought home a set of [BiomagScience] BioMagnets and applied them on him. I told him that this was much safer for his body since the magnets are applied externally.

He has been on Daytime and Nightime therapy since December 1995 (written in 1996). The results: I'd say quite satisfactory because his intake of medication has been reduced to once a day and he hasn't suffered an attack since then." ~ E.L.M.T., M.D.

Diagnosis, Malignant Brain Tumor

I am the father of three children. My youngest is now two. When she was 6 months old, I was diagnosed with a malignant brain tumor with no options. I was given 2 months to live. My heart was heavy and I was depressed. A friend asked me if I wanted to meet people who were involved with alternative healing. I thought to myself, what do I have to lose?

That meeting changed my life. I met Peter Kulish, founder of BiomagScience. He immediately prescribed a BioMagnetic therapy plan that included Meridian Energizing Therapy, Daytime Sternum Therapy and Nightime Therapy. I drank Bio-Negative Water, took Stabilized Oxygen (BAO), changed my eating habits and added colloidal minerals to my diet. I was determined to get well.

It's over a year later now and all traces of the tumor are gone. Today I am cancer-free. I live in Malaysia with my beautiful wife and children and work for the [Biomag Science] company that is dedicated to helping humanity. Thank you.   ~ R.L., Malaysia

Carpal Tunnel Syndrome Relieved

In 1994 I was diagnosed with carpal tunnel syndrome in my right hand. The pain was excruciating. I tried physical therapy, acupuncture, rest and a brace. Nothing helped. The pressure was too much. Within four years the pain had traveled up my arm. It was debilitating. I could no longer perform simple tasks such as lifting a book, writing or combing my hair.

I consulted a neurosurgeon for help. He said I had nerve damage and suggested surgery, as the only cure. Surgery didn't appeal to me and I felt there had to be something else that could help me.

Then I heard about BioMagnets. I wore the BioMagnets and within six days the pain that I had suffered with for four years was 80% better. Within 2 more weeks I was playing tennis. I know that sounds unbelievable, but it's true. I feel like a miracle happened for me. Thank you for helping my body heal in a natural way.

~ M. Rosensweet, CA

Splintered Broken Bones Heal in Several Months

A 73-year-old man was in a head-on collision just before Thanksgiving, which crushed both knees and splintered both legs down to his ankles. After surgery of screwing him back together, the doctor told him that he could expect to fully heal by August at which time he would start physiotherapy to learn how to walk again. Using Super magnets down the front of his left leg and the back of his right, he did not need any pain killers and was walking normally by the third week of January. So instead of healing in 10-12 months and having to re-learn to walk, he healed in just over a couple of months without pain pills and was able to walk almost immediately.

Awoken From Terminating Coma

A 91-year-old man's kidneys failed and his dialysis could no longer be done, so he slipped into a septic shock coma. Just before he was about to terminate, the Organ Group Energizing (OGE) therapy was applied and instead of terminating, he woke up and started healing. He lived on for approximately six months without the need of dialysis as his kidneys healed and functioned. Then he peacefully died in his sleep after indicating that he wanted to pass on to be with his wife who had died many years before. This case is responsible for the creation of the OGE therapy, which has been an extraordinary therapy in helping with cases of chronic illness.

Awoken From Terminating Coma

A middle-aged woman slipped into a coma from acute pancreatitis from a normal dose of antibiotics. With her vital signs indicating that she was going to terminate within a short period of time (possibly 2-3 days), the doctor indicated that her son could try "anything," so he put a Super BioMagnet over her pancreas and applied the MET (Meridian Energizing Therapy). Within three days, she awoke out of the coma and a week later, left the hospital fully healed – another profound reaction to advanced BiomagScience energy medicine.

Almost Quadriplegic, Paraplegic Man Walks Again

A 47-year-old man lost control of his motorcycle badly injuring his spine, breaking one of his legs and several ribs, leaving him paralyzed, unable to ever walk again. The nerve damage was so severe he could barely use his arms. He was in such pain that he had to use a morphine pump. After visiting over 20 doctors throughout the US who could not help him, he tried BiomagScience.

He took to the magnets with great interest and started with three METs (Meridian Energy Therapy) daily. He also slept with magnets religiously placed on the sternum and pineal gland [Nightime]. In addition, he drank at least 8 to 10 glasses of Bio-Negative energized water every day.

By the end of three months he began to notice some feeling coming back into his legs, arms and hands. At this point, he still could not shake hands with me. His pains had subsided somewhat, but he continued to use the morphine pump.

He was religious in using the magnets and was dedicated to continuing on with the Meridian Energy Therapy. By the fourth month, he could sit up and do some writing with his hands. By the seventh month, he began to walk and had regained enough strength to look forward to regaining a normal life. However, he still had limited mobility, some aches and pain and continued with the morphine pump.

By the tenth month, he was able to walk to a car and sit up; most of his pain had subsided enough to remove the pump. Within in a year he was brave enough to climb aboard a "Segway" motor bike and take it out for a ride. Six months following this, he actually stood up on his Segway motor bike and drove two miles up curvy roads in the hills in Santa Barbara to show off his returned health and well-being.

This man has normal health again and is back to running his business and leading a normal life.

Separated Nerve Regenerated in Knee

A nerve in the knee of a 72-year-old man was severed during surgery. His doctor said, "You will never feel anything below the knee ever again." The man reported to us, "Walking is extremely hard without feeling. I used the BiomagScience knee circuit therapy and the nerve was healed in less than a month. I'm now walking normally."

~ I. Ren.

Bedridden for 25 years, Woman Starts to Heal in an Hour

A middle-aged woman had chronic malabsorption, constipation, fibromyalgia and depression. Over the 25 year period, she had tried every allopathic and alternative therapy, including useless magnets, and nothing helped. Her vitality was so low that any supplement she took would act as a toxin and upset her as a toxic event.

Within one hour of BiomagScience CVS therapy, she started healing. The correct energy supplementation energized and restarted her cells, helping her overcome the malabsorption and start functioning normally. Within a year, she was playing competitive tennis and fully had her life back.

Rare Blind Eye Disease of Infant Resolved in 3 weeks

At 3 months, an infant was diagnosed as having manifest nystagmus with strabismus. Nystagmus means that the infant's eyes go from side to side and up and down continuously, not able to focus; if it is manifest, it is very aggressive (rapid) and if they have Strabismus, their eyes move independently, crossing over each other.

This condition creates blindness because the eyes cannot land to focus. Considered a fault in the neural system, including the cerebellovestibular, optokinetic and pursuit mechanisms that normally hold the eye's fixation (focus) steady, there was no known allopathic therapy to help the condition. Once the condition was established, Bio-Negative energy was applied on the top middle forehead to stimulate the frontal lobe where the hypotrophic [non-matured] area was considered to be. In 3 weeks, there were no longer any physical signs of involuntary and uncoordinated eye movements and the child started to see; the hypotrophic area's growth had caught up. After the 3 weeks, the biomagnet was moved up higher on the forehead every couple of weeks until it reached the top of the head.

No More Backache

Two years ago, I suffered from severe backache. The pain would occur every time my workload got heavy. One day, I attended a seminar on BioMagnetics. Hoping to solve my problem, I borrowed a set of BioMagnets and placed them over the affected area. I waited overnight for the results. The following day my back pain was gone. I was cured and impressed to say the least.

I also drank Negative Energized Water to supplement the therapy. From that time on, I haven't complained about my back pain. Now I am really determined to use a whole set, not only for my family, but also to help those who wish to be relieved of any illness.

~ Mrs. E. Capoy

Instant Relief from Asthma

I have proven for myself the effectiveness of [BiomagScience] BioMagnets. One time when I was having a bad asthma attack, I placed a [Super] BioMagnet on my sternum and immediately felt relief. Unlike drugs, that took many agonizing minutes before I felt better, the magnets worked instantly. I told myself that if I ever felt uneasy about pain or any disease that came my way, the answer would be BioMagnets.   ~ Mr. A. Martinez

I Couldn't Believe it

At first, I couldn't believe that this little device called a BioMagnet could heal any illness. Eventually, however, I became convinced about the healing power of [BiomagScience] BioMagnets. I had a toothache; out of curiosity I placed the magnet on my jaw where the aching tooth was. Just like some sort of magic, the pain disappeared within exactly five minutes. One time after that, I tried it for a headache. It also disappeared after a few minutes. These experiences totally convinced me that BioMagnets indeed can do healing wonders for any kind of disease.   ~ Ms. A. Mongas

Rodeo Injury Relieved

I was suffering constant pain in my right wrist due to a rodeo accident when I was 27 years old. I am now 54 years old, and until I discovered the healing power of BioMagnets, I had periodic swelling and pain in the wrist. I applied the magnets as per instructions and wore them for five days during the daytime. I noticed within the first hour that there was no pain in my wrist when I was wearing the magnets. By the second day, the swelling started to subside. The entire healing process took seven days and I now work normally at any task including typing at the computer. I still have slight wrist pain every few days, but when I place my magnets on the injured area for about one hour, the pain ends.

I have told many of my friends about BioMagnets and I will continue to do so in the coming years, as I have experienced the success story of BioMagnets for healing.   ~ R. Smith

Please see further case studies, testimonials, health conditions and research at www.BiomagScience.Net

Testimonials and case studies are inspirational true stories and studies that give hope to long-term sufferers of pain, illness and disease. When using magnets to assist the body in healing, there are always many factors that should be taken into consideration.

For example, while BioMagnets have been shown to provide fast relief from headaches, it may require additional therapy for migraines; it may be necessary to increase therapy time and drink BNW (Bio-Negative) energized water to overcome any dehydration and increase cellular function. It also may require CVS, MET & OGE therapies to help overcome the issue.

It is important to realize that factors such as stress, environmental toxicity, diet, and older physical injuries might be the culprits behind your discomfort. Using the process of elimination, take a look at your surroundings and ask yourself questions like the following: Are there toxic or noxious fumes in my environment? How close am I to my computer and other appliances that give off strong electric fields? Do I need to change my diet? When do I get my headaches? Is it in the morning when I wake up or is it when I'm at work?

In other words, your body provides the answers. In most cases, BioMagnetic therapies can help most health conditions if the protocols are applied completely for the full therapy period. Overcoming pain and rapid supportive healing is the common result from BiomagScience therapy.

Whenever in doubt, contact BiomagScience at Office@ BiomagScience.Net and they will help guide you.

CHAPTER FOURTEEN

MAGNETO–DIAGNOSTICS

Magneto-Diagnostics is a useful practitioner's diagnostic tool for measuring and determining the therapy for dysfunctioning glands and organs. An easy test to conduct, a SUPER BioMagnet is applied over each gland/organ to see if there is a kinesiologic (muscle) reaction to either the Negative or Positive magnetic field. If it reacts to one of the fields, then the opposite field is applied for 20 minutes as therapy to help normalize the condition. Then it is re-tested and re-applied for another 20 minutes as necessary.

Magneto-Diagnostics works by magnetically activating and measuring the reaction of the hydrogen ions in the gland/organ. If there is no reaction to both fields, the gland/organ is functioning properly. If there is a reaction, the gland/organ is dysfunctional and needs therapy. The Negative field is the most common response indicating a hypo-active gland/organ dysfunction (hydrogen ion deficiency). The Positive field indicates a hyper-active function (excess of hydrogen ions).

Magneto-Diagnostic Procedure

Using the testing technique on the next page, apply the Super BioMagnet Negative and then Positive on each gland and organ. Record any reaction in the chart that follows (Positive/Negative).

Therapy: Apply a 2-stack of Regulars (on the organs) or Power Wafers (on the glands) of the field opposite to the test reaction on the affected glands or organs for 20 minutes; and then,

Retest, record and re-apply the required therapy field for another 20 minutes if required. Send client home with Daytime, Nightime Biomagnets and BAO (BiomagScience Activated Oxygen).

Testing Procedure

If another type of kinesiologic tool is used, it may not require two practitioners or caregivers. The following Magneto-Diagnostics kinesiologic testing uses two people: One practitioner/caregiver holding the legs for the reaction and the other testing each organ/gland with both poles of the Super BioMagnet.

Testing the Client

Lay the person down on his/her back with the legs over the end of the table. One practitioner/caregiver holds the legs about 6" in the air while the other practitioner places the Super BioMagnet on the skin over each gland/organ, first Negative, then Positive. If there is a reaction to the Testing Magnet, a spasmodic involuntary jerk of the leg(s) will be felt by the practitioner. This is a kinesiologic response to that specific gland or organ.

No reaction: the gland/organ is functioning correctly.
Negative field reaction: hypo-active dysfunctioning state.
Positive field reaction: hyper-active dysfunctioning state.

Record the reaction of each gland/organ in the following chart. The chart lists each organ tested, the date, and reaction of two concurrent tests. See pgs. 155-156 for BioMagnet placement location.

Therapy

Apply the opposite magnetic field to the gland/organ test response area for 20 minutes. For example:

Apply the Positive field to help normalize a Negative hypo-active gland/organ to a healthy state; and/or,

Apply the Negative field to help normalize a Positive hyper-active gland/organ to a healthy state.

Recommended During Therapy

It is recommended that a 2-Stack of Power Wafers Bio-Negative be placed over the sternum (♥PD WARNING, p. 117) during the therapy period to ensure the body is systemically receiving Bio-Negative healing energy.

Therapy Time

The normal therapy period is 20 minutes. Each hypo- or hyper-active organ/gland receives a 20-minute therapy with the opposite polarity of the test reaction. Therapy can be applied at the same time on all organs/glands that reacted to the fields.

After the 20 minutes, repeat the test and apply the therapy for any glands/organs needing further energy work. It may be required to do the therapy every 3 days for 3 or more times, as indicated by the progress. The Practitioner should test and chart the reactions each time to notate the progress. See illustration pgs. 155-156.

It is important that the client continue with energy supplementation during and after the Magneto-Diagnostic therapy sessions with the Daytime and Nightime therapies, Bio-Negative energized water and any BiomagScience Activated Oxygen as recommended. See acute illness or chronic conditions, p. 108.

Testing chart follows below. Copy as needed.

Name			Date	
Organ	**Test 1**(reaction only) -+ **Comment**		**Test 2** (reaction only) -+ **Comment**	
Pineal				
Thymus				
Thyroid				
Parathyroid				
Lung Right				
Left				
Heart				
Liver				
Gallbladder				
Spleen				
Pancreas				
Kidney Right				
Left				
Stomach				
Large Intestine				
Small Intestine				
Ovaries				
Uterus				
Testes				
Comments				

Magneto-Diagnostics Client Positioning

1. Place person on back holding legs in a relaxed position.
2. Test client by placing Super BioMagnet on gland/organ, first Negative and then Positive.
3. Watch for and record reaction.
4. Apply therapy on each gland/organ with the opposite magnetic polarity to the reaction for 20 minutes.
5. Re-test and record results.
6. Re-Apply therapy on each gland/organ with the opposite magnetic polarity to the reaction for 20 minutes.
7. Repeat therapy every 3 days for a total of 3-4 therapies.

♥PD WARNING for any sternum placement

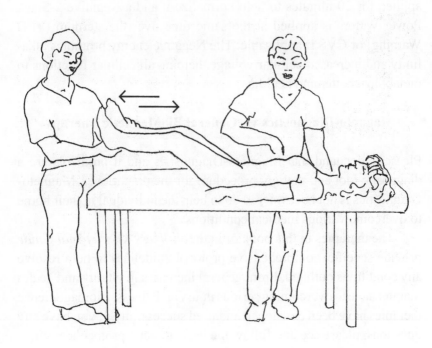

Acute, Chronic Conditions

If the medical condition is acute or chronic, it is suggested that the ATACC (acute chronic therapy protocols) in the *Wellness Kit Pictorial Guide* be applied immediately to energize and rebalance the biochemistry to help quickly return to health. These will include the OGE (Organ Group Energizing) therapy, MET (Meridian Energizing Therapy), Daytime, Nightime, Bio-Negative water and Activated Oxygen Therapies to help the body rapidly return to health.

Please note and REMEMBER, whenever the Positive application is being applied whether separately or in a Circuit, it is important to use Negative BioMagnet concurrently on the sternum (♥PD WARNING p. 117) or lower CVS to ensure the body is receiving an adequate amount of healing Bio-Negative energy, especially when the Positive therapy is required.

For example: If a liver is hypo-active, the Positive pole is applied for 20 minutes to help normalize it and a Negative 2-Stack Power Wafers is applied at the same time over the sternum (♥PD Warning) or CVS if applicable. The Negative energy promotes alkalinity and increased cellular voltage, helping all cellular functions to metabolize better and healthier.

Magneto-Diagnostics vs. General BioMagnetic Therapy

Please understand that Magneto-Diagnostics and it protocols are a diagnostic tool and therapy procedure for the practitioner. Magneto-Diagnostics is not necessary to do to help the individual in their home to overcome various medical conditions.

The therapies in this book or in the *Wellness Kit Pictorial Guide* provide specific, comprehensive protocol guidelines to help resolve any conditions outlined. From general increases in vitality and health maintenance to overcoming serious injury and illness, BiomagScience therapies have been developed and used successfully. If you have any questions, please see and follow the basic therapy protocols outlined in Chapters 15 through 18.

SECTION 2

HOW TO USE BIOMAGNETIC THERAPIES

This section of the book includes instructions on how to specifically use BioMagnetic therapies for energizing the body to help it heal rapidly. It is important to read all the directions before starting. Make note of the following:

- BiomagScience Certified BioMagnets are universally marked either green (-) Negative or red (+) Positive and have raised letters on the Positive side so the polarity can be checked by touch when applying them out of sight, such as on the back.
- The body diagrams are shown in anatomical position with the arms down along the leg and the palm forward with thumbs out perpendicular from the side of the leg. The anatomical viewpoint is used to indicate the proper meridian placement as shown in the Proper Polarity Placement, p. 138.

To Begin BioMagnetic Therapy Protocols

- Read BioMagnetic Precautions and Basics before starting any procedure.
- Be aware of the ♥PD WARNING sign (Pacemaker/Defibrillator Warning, p. 117).
- Familiarize yourself with BiomagScience Products, Therapy Techniques, Abbreviations, Proper Polarity Placement and Illustrations.
- Look up the therapy for an ailment listed alphabetically in Health Conditions and BioMagnetic Therapies.
- For detailed information on the BioMagnets or products used in this book, see the *BiomagScience Product Information* section near the end of the book.

Come join us online at our "BiomagScience Medical Magnet Forum" at MagneticTherapyToday@YahooGroups.com, where we answer your health questions about magnetic therapy.

CHAPTER FIFTEEN

BASIC BIOMAGNETIC THERAPY AND PRECAUTIONS

Bio-Negative North Pole Healing Energy

When the body is healthy, the cells have a natural alkaline Negative mV (millivoltage) charge. Whenever painful inflammation occurs from infection, stress, trauma, injury or illness, the damaged cells healthy Negative mV is reduced, their immune functions are impaired, and they move toward a slightly Positive acid state. As a result, the brain immediately floods the site with healing Negative energy to increase the cellular mV and immune functions. This is why Bio-Negative (Geo North) energy is the primary therapy energy used to help the body heal rapidly – because it amplifies and super-charges the body's own natural healing energy. See "Therapy Protocols," p. 136.

Bio-Negative energy also works as an antioxidant (Negative charged donor electrons), neutralizing the Positively charged oxidative free-radicals while increasing the Negative cellular voltage and immune functions which help the damaged cells heal rapidly. Please see www. BiomagScience.Net before and after free-radical test research.

Daily Bio-Negative energy supplementation (Daytime therapy) provides a high state of cellular voltage and vitality throughout the body which supports and maintains good health, wellness and is a natural defense against free-radicals and illness.

Proper Polarity Placement: Each side of the limb, hip or shoulder has a Positive and Negative side (p. 126) and application of the Bio-Negative energy must be on the Negative meridian side.

The exception of placing Bio-Negative on a Positive Meridian for twenty minutes is for short-term topical issues only, such as burns, cuts, cysts or insect bites, where a single Power Wafer is used.

All Bio-Negative skin applications for *non-topical*, penetrating tissue therapy on a Positive Meridian can cause electromotive stress which increases pain and does not provide healing.

In other words, if it is for any kind of skin condition, it is alright to use a single Power Wafer Bio-Negative anywhere, but if it is therapy for any tissue below the skin anywhere on the limb, the Bio-Negative must be placed on the Negative meridian, not the Positive. Please review the Proper Polarity Placement chapter before applying therapy on a limb, shoulder, or hip.

Pain relief from Bio-Negative therapy generally occurs within minutes to several hours of application; in acute/chronic cases, it may require up to 3 days to achieve relief from pain. After achieving pain relief, the application should be continued for another 7-10 days to ensure the healing is complete; otherwise it may return.

If there is no relief after 3 days, apply the "Circuit Therapy," p 147 or in the Wellness Kit Pictorial Guide which helps reduce pain by regenerating the missing or worn out soft and/or hard tissue, including severed nerves, connective tissue, cartilage, vertebrae, bad back, sciatica, fractures, rotator cuff, or joints such as elbow, knee, or hip. (See Chapter 13, "Testimonials/Case Studies," and "Health Conditions and Research" at www.BiomagScience.Net.)

Any inflammation/fluid-buildup that has not responded to Negative energy in 3 days requires moving the BioNegative BioMagnet 3 inches in the direction toward the heart. Once the fluid is reduced, reapply the BioMagnet over the site to help it rapidly heal.

Positive South Pole Energy

The Bio-Positive energy should only be used as directed by your practitioner, or as instructed in this book and in BiomagScience Kits. The Positive energy can over-stimulate and stress the metabolism; it is used safely by the practitioner in organ/gland therapy and in conjunction with the Bio-Negative in Circuit Therapies such as the MET (Meridian Energizing Therapy), for Back, Carpal Tunnel, etc. in which the Negative directs the Positive energy into a safe, profound healing configuration.

Using the Positive energy separately without Negative energy control can create oxidation, acidosis, stress, inflammation, tumors, increased anaerobic [bad] bacteria and metabolic hyperactivity, leading to further health issues. BiomagScience has found its use in the advanced Circuit Therapy Protocols to be completely safe and has produced profound results in nerve and tissue regeneration never seen or experienced before.

Positive Energy Field – Use the Bio-Positive (+) red side

- Complete System Energizing & Balancing with the MET (Meridian Energizing Therapy) used with the Negative energy.

- Bone, Cartilage & Nerve Regeneration/reunion used with the Bio-Negative in Circuit Therapy.

Always make sure that the Positive is applied on the Positive Polarity Meridian of the limbs (see p. 138) and the *Quick Reference Guide* on p. ix.

Magnetic Foot Pad Inserts – Caution Please

Research indicates that both monopolar and bipolar footpads *initially* provide a good feeling as they help resolve MDS (Magnetic Deficiency Syndrome). Days later, however, subtle, detrimental changes can occur elsewhere in the body as a result of using the pads.

Energy medicine disciplines of Shiatsu, Acupuncture and Reflexology teach that the trigger points in the feet affect specific glands/organs/muscles. Research has shown that Negative or Positive magnetism under a trigger point can cause hypo or hyperactivity in the associated gland/organ/muscle. Example: a fellow, after asking whether the magnetic foot pad would affect his pacemaker, had to remove it immediately because his pacemaker became erratic.

BiomagScience *does not recommend* wearing magnetic foot pads, or at best, *for not much longer than 3-5 days* to avoid improper hypo- or hyperactive stimulation of vital organ/gland/muscle functions that could adversely affect your health and vitality. *As a precaution, use Daytime Sternum Therapy while wearing magnetic foot pads.* (See "Circulation and Feet," Chapter 20.)

Magnetic Beds or Mattress Pads – Caution Please

Magnetic beds or mattress pads should be used with caution. Do not buy multi-polar beds as they emit Positive energy which is bad for you. Many companies sell these pads/beds without explaining that at first, the magnetic system may feel good as it helps reduce MDS. However, continued use of the Positive energy from the bi-polar field will reduce cellular energy, creating inflammation, pain, dysfunction, acidosis, and immune system failure leading to illness and disease.

BiomagScience worked with an individual who had a bad magnetic bed. One of her friends had brought her to see if we could help her. Her pain was so intense she was suicidal, so someone would have to be with her all the time. Consulting with her, we were able to isolate the problem as being a bad magnetic bed she had purchased from the Japanese magnetic company, Nikken. She had never suspected the bed was the cause of her pain, because when she first used it she felt better. She didn't know that lying on Positive energy all night was inflaming her body and creating pain. We advised she stop sleeping on it and start Bio-Negative therapy immediately; she did and within days, the pain was relieved and within weeks, she became healthy again.

Subsequently that company finally started promoting its Negative-only beds. We learned this from an individual who felt a bit strange after buying one that upon testing with our medical magnets, we found that there were quite a few magnets that were Positive. So be very careful in acquiring a properly made magnetic bed or pad for sleeping on.

Pregnancy – Caution

While one is pregnant, it is advised not to use BioMagnets directly over the womb or lower torso of the body, as the direct energy may interfere with the growth of the fetus. The Daytime, CVS, Nightime, and Bio-Negative water therapies do not interfere with the fetus, but provide supplemental energy to both the mother and the fetus.

Biomagnet Daily Energy Supplementation
Daytime (sternum) Therapy

The sternum/heart is the primary energizing point of the body and this therapy is the one most used to increase cellular energy to help heal an injury or medical condition and is used for maintaining wellness and vitality. As the heart pumps, the healing Negative energy goes into the heart and blood and throughout the body.

Daytime Therapy

Daily, people all over the world use the Daytime therapy to stay healthy and energetic. Applied in the morning all day till bedtime, a 2-Stack of PWs (Power Wafers) is applied Bio-Negative green over the indentation of the sternum/breastbone, one inside and one outside the shirt/blouse or center bra strap to hold each other in place. If the PWs on the bra strap are too far away from the sternum, place them just inside and outside the left bra cup next to the center strap.

If you catch a cold or virus and need extra energy to help overcome it, apply a 2-Stack of Regulars to increase the energy.

Nausea at First with the Daytime Therapy

Some individuals who have had very low energy or have been sick for some time may experience nervousness and possible nausea when first using the Daytime Therapy. This reaction indicates that the cells are energizing and starting to detoxify very rapidly (Herxheimer effect). Normally after a period of low cellular vitality/voltage, the toxins build up in the cells. When the cellular energy is increased, the toxins are naturally eliminated as the cell normalizes.

The toxic elimination period normally lasts for 4-10 hours. If it is too uncomfortable and you want to bypass the heavy detoxification, move the Negative 2-Stack PWs from the sternum and place them on the lower CVS (cerebral vestibular system – middle back of the neck on the skin at the hairline) for an hour the first day, increasing it an hour more each day until the 5th day, when you should be able to apply the Daytime sternum placement without experiencing any nausea.

Degenerative Heart Condition

Heart Problem Warning: If a degenerative heart problem exists, do not use the Daytime sternum placement. Use the safe lower CVS (cerebral vestibular system – middle back of the neck on the skin at the hairline) placement. Apply the Negative (-) 2-Stack PWs green side on the skin. Most people either use a band-aid between the PWs or place one inside and one outside the collar to hold each other in place.

Pacemaker/Defibrillator ♥PD WARNING

Do not use a magnetic field within 8 inches of a defibrillator or pacemaker. The magnetic field can disrupt the functioning of these appliances and slow down or stop the device. If the therapy indicates the Daytime (sternum) Placement and there is a heart appliance, it has been found that the 2-Stack Power Wafers, Negative green side on lower CVS (middle back of the neck on skin at the hairline) is safe.

Do Not Use magnetic foot pads or mattresses with a pacemaker or defibrillator, as the trigger point for the heart in the foot has been shown to sometimes cause an electrical dysfunction in the device. A mattress can cause an electrical dysfunction in the device.

Circulation Blood Pressure and Diabetes

Circulation can be stimulated by the Negative pole, which can help soften the hardening of the vascular system. The Negative energy increases the blood cell energy (Zeta potential) which breaks up the hypercoagulation Rouleau pattern of the blood cells clustering together. The clustered cells can increase the formation of plaque, which puts one at risk for heart attack and stroke. The increased Zeta potential also reduces abnormally high calcium ions, resulting in plaque reduction and increased circulation. See *Natural Blood Thinner*, p. 166.

BiomagScience Circulation Enzymes is an oral chelation supplement. When taken daily with Biomagnetic energy supplementation, it has been shown not only to reduce vascular plaque, but with the energy therapy, it reduces cellular plaque.

A 3-month therapy term of Circulation Enzymes, Daytime Therapy and Bio-Negative energized water has been shown repeatedly to normalize high BP (blood pressure), eliminating the need for BP medicine; eliminate major plaque buildup such as arterial stenosis; and resolve dark-colored feet and peripheral neuropathy due to poor circulation.

Diabetes

Many Type II diabetic individuals doing the 3-month therapy overcame their diabetes as the plaque was eliminated from their pancreatic cells and their metabolic functions were normalized.

Always Be Careful with Your Biomagnets

They can demagnetize your credit cards, tapes and other magnetic surfaces. Keep at least 3-4 inches from any surface that would be affected by the magnetism including but not limited to computers, smart phones, etc.

CHAPTER SIXTEEN

RESPONSE OF THE MAGNETIC POLES

THE NORTH (Geological) BIO-NEGATIVE POLE

Green is the universal BioMagnetic color for Bio-Negative energy. The Negative field is the primary healing energy and provides the following:

- Sedates nerve tissue to reduce and inhibit pain.
- Reduces/eliminates inflammation/pain to support rapid healing.
- Normalizes cellular voltage, increasing cellular transfer efficiency of oxygen, nutrition and detoxification for improved metabolic and immune functions for healing and maintaining wellness.
- Slows down and normalizes hyperactive organs and glands.
- Helps control coagulation of bleeding of wounds at an injury site.
- Vasodilates constricted tissue.
- Natural blood thinner: increased blood cell energy (Zeta potential) breaks up the dangerous Rouleau pattern, the clumping of blood cells known as hypercoagulation, which creates plaque-building often responsible for heart attack and stroke.
- Helps reduce buildup of fatty-deposits and plaque in veins/arteries.
- Arresting effect on anaerobic bacteria and aberrant growths.
- Decreases abnormal calcium ions; helps direct minerals to target sites.
- Helps normalize gene transcription, which helps overcome certain genetic issues by reducing bridge lengths between gene transmitter and receptor sites and increasing neural amplitude. This results in more complete genetic code transmission.

The negative (-), North side of the magnet is the pole most frequently used for healing. It is very important to health. Trauma causes the cellular condition to go into a positive acid state. The negative pole will increase alkalinity and reduce acidity. It decreases acidity in ailments by reducing the hydrogen ion, increasing pH and causing alkalinity to bring the tissue back to normal. Alkalinity fights colds, bacteria and increases oxygen to the cell.

Summary Bio-Negative Pole

The Bio-Negative (-) energy is used most frequently in healing therapies. It amplifies the body's own natural Negative healing energy, which provides pain relief, healing of injuries, and increased immune function for fighting colds, bacteria, overcoming illness/disease, and providing daily wellness and vitality.

Trauma causes the cells/tissue to go into a slight Positive acid state. The Bio-Negative energy supports the rapid healing of traumatized cells/tissue by increasing and normalizing their weakened energy. This increases the pH, causing the cells/ tissue to alkalize and increase hydration, cellular oxygenation, nutrition, detoxification, and immune functions for rapid pain relief and healing.

When the body is hurt, a signal is sent to the brain which sends a signal to flood the area with Negative charges to heal it. The Bio-Negative energy substantially amplifies the healing energy for quick pain relief and healing.

The Bio-Negative energy is used for aches, pains, inflammation, arthritis, bleeding, wounds, sores, boils, eczema, skin rashes, burns, infections, toothache, kidney infection, kidney stones, cancer (helps sedate the pain, arrest and alkalize the condition), bladder complaints and most medical conditions. The Bio-Negative energy is also used with the Bio-Positive energy for advanced Circuit Therapies for chronic illness and regeneration of nerve and soft and hard tissue.

THE SOUTH (Geological) BIO-POSITIVE POLE

Red is the universal biomagnetic color for Bio-Positive energy. Positive energy stimulates all forms of life including anaerobic bacteria – do not use unless specified by therapies in this book, in a Circuit Therapy or as indicated in the *Wellness Kit Pictorial Guide* or by a BiomagScience practitioner.

- Stimulates activity in the glands/organs in its energy field by attracting and increasing hydrogen ions in glands or organs.
- Long term use can cause acidosis/illness; short-term: neutralizes stomach acidity; in the colon, increases peristalsis to relieve constipation.
- Increases infection, anaerobic bacteria and aberrant cell growth.
- Expands and enlarges tissue by increasing inter/intracellular fluids (in and around the cells), Used in back therapy with Bio-Negative energy to reduce and eliminate pain.
- Can constrict circulation by increasing inflammation – do not use on inflammation.
- Can create additional bleeding when there is a cut or abrasion.

Summary Bio-Positive Pole

The Bio-Positive energy is used to quickly neutralize stomach acid, increase peristalsis (muscle action of colon) to help overcome constipation; in magneto-diagnostics, as therapy to overcome hypoactive gland and organ functions. The Bio-Positive energy is used as an integral part of the Positive/Negative energy placement in all Circuit Therapies to reduce pain and help regenerate and heal connective, nerve, and soft and hard tissue for injury, trauma, non-union fractures, severed nerves, worn out joints, and acute medical conditions. The Positive is used in a circuit with the Negative energy in the MET (Meridian Energizing Therapy) to energize and balance the entire body to help overcome chronic illness/disease and the BRT (Brain

Re-Entrainment Therapy) for visual (optokinetic), neurological (post stroke, etc.) and bio-chemically unstable mental conditions. See Chapter 18.

CHAPTER SEVENTEEN

THE BASICS

BiomagScience BioMagnets are the most powerful, state of the art medical magnets available anywhere and are certified by the Foundation for Magnetic Science. They come in three different sizes to fulfill the power that is required for the therapy. They are color-coded with raised letters on the Positive Red side so the proper polarity can be felt when applying them out of sight, such as on the back.

BiomagScience BioMagnets can be applied to the body with medical tape, band-aids, bandages and often on both sides of the clothing, band-aid, or tape to hold each other in place in a 2-Stack (stack of two) configuration.

Unless the extremely powerful Super Biomagnet is required, the 2-Stack of Power Wafers or Regulars is specially designed to provide the depth and width of energy penetration for the required therapy and can be worn discreetly without cumbersome, hot, sweaty application devices.

BiomagScience Rare Earth BioMagnets Come in Three Sizes.
See p. 38 for power and penetration measurements.

- **PW** (Power Wafer): Topical Lite/Wide Field, 3" AF (Active Field)
- **2-Stack PWs**: Medium Lite/Wide Field, 4" AF
- **RB (Regular)**: Medium Deep/Wide Field, 10" AF
- **2-Stack RBs**: Very Deep/Wide Field, 18" AF
- **Super**: Very Deep/Wide, 22" AF

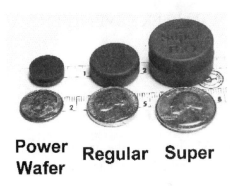

Power Wafer   **Regular**   **Super**

BiomagScience Health Products

Power Wafer BioMagnet ("PW"): For general pain and vitality; about the size of a dime, lightweight, very powerful and easy to apply; excellent for most areas of pain and healing. When used as a single PW application for skin conditions (bite, burn, scrape, baker's cyst, etc.), it may be applied anywhere. The PW are often used in stack of two known as a "2-Stack PWs" for general pain relief and to help healing. When a 2-Stack PWs are applied on the limbs, they are always placed to conform to the Proper Polarity Placement (PPP, p. 138) of the limb's meridian.

The 2-Stack PWs is commonly used on the sternum (Daytime therapy) or lower CVS (back of the neck) for improving general health and maintaining wellness.

Regular BioMagnet ("RB"): Used for medium deep and wide tissue penetration for pain relief and healing support; in a 2-Stack for very deep, wide penetration for powerful healing support; and in "Circuit Therapies" (p.147 and in the *Wellness Kit Pictorial Guide*) to help regenerate connective tissue, nerves, bones, joints, back, etc.

The Regulars are used in the MET (Meridian Energizing Therapy, p.131) for energizing and balancing the biochemistry and stimulating the nervous system for healing and wellness. This is an important advanced therapy that has created miracle-like results. These are used also for the OGE (Organ Group Energizing) therapy which uniformly energizes the primary organs to fully function including full enzymatic and hormonal outputs to overcome extremely acute and chronic illness.

Super BioMagnet ("Super"): Our most powerful BioMagnet; for wide area, very deep tissue therapy for glands/organs and advanced chronic illness. Extremely powerful, the Super's field reaches 22" and is used for deep and/or aberrant tissue conditions.

Bio-Negative Water ("BNW") Jar Magnets / Under-the-Sink Cold-Water-Line Energizer: An inexpensive system for a lifetime of healthy, Negatively charged water. Simply attaches to the outside of a water container or under the sink. See Chapter 7.

BiomagScience Activated Oxygen ("BAO"): One of the safest forms of oxygen in liquid, for use in **BNW** internal/external therapies. Used to increase metabolic functions, it is also used to overcome burns, scrapes, colds, viruses, anaerobic bacteria, help heal illness and maintain wellness. See Chapter 8 for use/dosage.

Ultimate Supplement ("hGH"): A naturally-derived liquid bio-identical hGH (human Growth Hormone) supplement to assist in healing, immune functions, new cell division, anti-aging, increased energy/vitality, and better sleeping; used to overcome chronic illness.

Circulation Enzymes ("CE"): An oral chelation that increases circulation, such as black feet, by eliminating plaque in the vascular system (veins and arteries), which also helps to lower blood pressure and normalize cholesterol.

When used with daily energy (Daytime) therapy, helps to eliminate plaque in the cells and has helped resolve Type II diabetes in numerous cases; often used in acute and chronic medical conditions.

Typical cases: eliminated arterial stenosis (plaque/calcium) buildup in the heart of middle-aged female within 6 weeks. 72-year-old male blood pressure went from 160/140 to 117/75 in three months.

General BioMagnet Directions

Examples of Therapy Techniques

First, BioMagnets are very easy to use and apply by taping the appropriate Negative green or Positive red side against the skin with a band-aid, medical tape, or bandage. Or one can often use a 2-Stack of BioMagnets placing both BioMagnets on both sides of the band-aid, tape, bandage or clothing to help hold each other in place.

Directions are always given to apply either the "Negative" (green) or "Positive" (red) side of the BioMagnet facing the skin/body. These directions will specify which size of the BioMagnet (PW-Power Wafer, RB-Regular BioMagnet or Super BioMagnet) to use and whether it is a 2-Stack and where to apply it.

"2-Stack" means 2 Biomagnets stacked on top of each other with a band-aid, bandage, medical tape or clothing in-between, such as:

- **2-Stack PWs** (Power Wafers)
- **2-Stack RBs** (Regular Biomagnets)
- **2-Stack PW/RB** (Power Wafer & Regular Biomagnet)

ATACC –Acute Chronic Therapy Protocols: Some acute and chronic (long term illness, CFS, Fibromyalgia, MS, etc.) medical conditions will require the advanced step-by-step therapies of the ATACC in the Wellness Kit Pictorial Guide. The ATACC requires most of the various-sized BioMagnets, Water Jar Magnets, and BAO (BiomagScience Activated Oxygen) in the BiomagScience Wellness Kit.

BAO: Many therapies require BAO (BiomagScience Activated Oxygen) mixed in with BNW (Bio-Negative Water). This provides increased blood oxygen percentage needed for healthy metabolism and increased energy. (See Chapter 8.)

Pain Therapy Example: Negative 2-Stack PWs or 2-Stack RBs, or 2-Stack PW/RB is placed on pain site – the BioMagnet size/configuration is dependent upon the depth of tissue penetration that is required. For skin condition placement, see p. 143. For non-skin tissue therapy on the limbs and extremities, always make sure the Negative green is applied on the Negative Meridian. (See PPP – Proper Polarity Placement, p.138.)

As noted in the PPP, if the pain is in the Positive meridian, apply the Bio-Negative green in the Negative meridian exactly opposite the pain so that the Negative healing energy follows the body's natural flow into the positive pain site. Term: apply until the pain stops.

Acne Example: Negative 2-stack PWs applied 30 minutes daily on area of outbreak. Wash with BNW (Bio-Negative Energized Water) and BAO (BiomagScience Activated Oxygen). Do the Daytime (♥PD WARNING), Nightime therapies. Drink BNW with BAO. Eliminate sugar and oily foods. Term: continuous.

Example 2 requires the reader to look up the dosage for BAO found in Chapter 8 – Activated Oxygen.

Chronic Fatigue Syndrome (CFS) Example: Apply the following ATACC (Acute Chronic Therapy Protocols) in the Wellness Book Pictorial Guide: OGE (Organ Group Energizing Therapy), MET (Meridian Energizing Therapy), Daytime (♥PD WARNING), Nightime. Drink BNW with BAO. Supplement hGH for 3 months. See *Nutrition*. See Medical Nutritionist. Term: 4 - 8 weeks.

In some therapies (such as example 3) it will be necessary for the reader to apply the therapies explained in the next chapter: Daytime and Nighttime Therapies, Organ Group Therapy, Meridian Energizing Therapy, Proper Polarity Placement and Circuit Therapy [Vortex Healing] therapy.

Therapy Acronyms and Abbreviations for therapies such as CVS & BAO are used for brevity and are on page 178. CVS, for example, stands for the *lower Cerebellar Vestibular System and is generally applied with a Negative 2-stack of PWs (Power Wafers) with a band-aid or on both sides of a shirt collar;* its abbreviation is on p.178 and in the *Glossary* with its definition and the location for magnetic placement (which is at the middle back of the neck at the hairline).

CHAPTER EIGHTEEN

BIOMAGNETIC THERAPY TECHNIQUES

A Must-Read chapter before applying the BioMagnets

This chapter describes the special therapies used in health conditions in Chapter 20, *Health Problems and BioMagnetic Therapies*

BiomagScience BioMagnets & Supplements used in therapies

- **PW** – Power Wafer BioMagnets
- **RB** – Regular BioMagnets
- **Super** – Super BioMagnet
- **BNW** – Bio-Negative Water
- **BAO** – BiomagScience Activated Oxygen
- **hGH** – Ultimate Supplement human Growth Hormone
- **CE** – Circulation Enzymes – oral chelation

Individual Therapies referenced:

- **Daytime** – Sternum/CVS Therapy for Health Maintenance
- **Nightime** – Nightime Therapy
- **OGE** – Organ Group Energizing Therapy
- **MET** – Meridian Energizing Therapy
- **PPP** – Proper Polarity Placement
- **CT** – Circuit Therapy (Vortex Initiation Healing Therapy)
- **BRT** – Brain Re-Entrainment Therapy
- **PPP** – Proper Polarity Placement

For BioMagnet applications, see *Illustrations,* 153, PPP, p. 138, *Quick Reference Guide* (p. ix) and *Wellness Kit Pictorial Guide.*

Basic BioMagnetic Therapy Techniques

For pain from injury, sprains, strains, joints, back or inflammation, a 2-Stack Bio-Negative field may be applied anywhere on the torso, but when applied on the shoulders and limbs, it must be placed in the Negative meridian to ensure the healing energy flows properly to help quickly resolve the issue without stress.

See *Proper Polarity Placement* (PPP, p. 138) or the Quick Reference Guide on p. ix for the correct applications for rapid pain relief and healing on the shoulders and limbs.

Example: the Bio-Negative can be applied directly on the front of the left leg over a torn meniscus, but if on the right leg, it must be applied on the back of the leg exactly opposite the meniscus.

Exception of Bio-Negative green on a Positive meridian: A single Power Wafer may be used for *20 Minutes ONLY* for a skin condition such as a burn, cut, scrape or baker's cyst. Remove after 20 minutes, as the area will become stressed and may start to hurt. Normally 20 minutes is enough time to start the healing of a skin condition.

Pain Relief: Most pain relief from therapy application occurs within minutes to hours, but may take up to 3.5 days to achieve comfort. If there is no relief after 3.5 days, then the Circuit Therapy will be required for pain relief/healing (p. 147 or in the *Wellness Kit Pictorial Guide*).

Basic and Advanced Therapies
Most are shown in the following illustrations.

Daytime (Sternum) Therapy Increases Energy & Wellness: The Daytime Sternum Therapy, also known as the "Daytime," uses a 2-Stack PWs Bio-Negative green over the indentation of the sternum

/breastbone. It is applied in the morning and worn till bedtime for full body energy supplementation. Most people wear them daily with a day off every so often when they instinctively feel they have had enough energy.

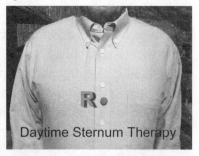
Daytime Sternum Therapy

If nervousness is felt when first using the Daytime therapy, reduce the power by moving the Bio-Negative green 2-Stack of PWs to the lower CVS (back of the neck on skin at hairline, pgs. 116, 178, 229) for 3-10 days until the Daytime can be worn without nervousness. **Warning: Do not apply Daytime therapy if you have a pacemaker/defibrillator. See ♥PD WARNING p. 117.**

Nightime Therapy Increases Energy & Wellness: Nightime Therapy, known as "Nightime," helps achieve deep, restorative sleep necessary for healing. As we age, the pineal gland often becomes hypoactive and does not produce enough melatonin to enable us to sleep well and heal. By applying a 2-Stack of PWs Bio-Negative green on the crown (top) of the head, the pineal gland is energized to put out a normal amount of melatonin for sleeping.

The Nightime Therapy is often used for 10 days to 3 weeks to retrain the pineal gland to normalize melatonin output. BiomagScience has clients who have worn it daily for several decades because it gives such great sleep and daily energy.

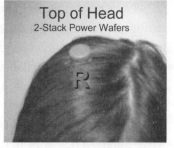
Top of Head
2-Stack Power Wafers

People often weave the 2-Stack PW into their hair by pulling the hair over the first PW and then placing the second over it to hold them both in place; women often use a barrette to hold the PWs, while others use a sleeping cap.

Meridian Energizing Therapy (MET): The MET was developed to overcome acute/chronic illness/disease by energizing and balancing the entire body so cellular functions would normalize and quickly heal. The MET [applied on the head, hands and feet] first energizes the cells in the central and peripheral nervous system, then expands the energy to the cells/tissue in the extremities and throughout the body. The MET quickly energizes the body's cells to help overcome long-term illness and disease.

Energizing the cells is like charging a car battery – when the battery is low, the lights, radio and engine can't operate correctly. When the body's cells are sick or hurt, their charge is low and their metabolic and immune functions cannot operate properly. Charging them with Bio-Negative energy helps raise their charge, which normalizes their functions, helps healing, and reduces pain.

Science teaches that energy always seeks balance. BiomagScience research has shown that the MET energy from the five peripheral points of the body travels to meet and balance at the solar plexus. During its travel, any weak, low-energy cells, such as in nerve, gland, organ or muscle tissue, that cannot carry (bridge) the energy forward are energized so they will bridge the energy and it can continue forward on its path to meet and balance. The energized formerly weak cells are now functioning and healthy.

The MET's ability to energize, balance and help heal is a major therapy breakthrough in helping overcome heretofore acute/chronic health issues that could not be addressed with allopathic medicine.

Examples of the MET are awakening an individual from a terminating coma, helping a quadriplegic regenerate his nerves for walking and living normally again, helping overcome 15- and 25- year bedridden, chronic malabsorption, and many other conditions too numerous to list.

Meridian Energizing Therapy Placement: Review the following MET diagram below or in the *Wellness Kit Pictorial Guide*. It is suggested that the MET be done when at rest either sitting or reclining.

Please Note: Any BioMagnet application directly in the MET circuit such as the lower CVS, spine, elbow, knee, etc. must be removed during the MET, as it interferes with the therapy. The Daytime and any organ therapies are not in the circuit and are OK.

- Apply Negative RB on the palm of left hand and right foot arch and Positive RB on the palm of right hand and left foot arch.

- Alternative MET hand & foot application: Use a bandage or wrap and apply the Negative RB on the wrist just above the palm of left-hand and the back of the ankle of the right foot; and put the Positive RB on the wrist just above the palm of right hand and on the back of the ankle of the left foot.

- Use 2-Stack Negative PW on crown of head.

- Do the Daytime (♥PD WARNING*) and continue after the MET.

- Drink Bio-Negative energized water with BAO to increase cellular nutrition/oxygen and detoxification.

- Therapy Term: 30-45 minutes daily for 10 days or as indicated by the condition's therapy. See Wellness Kit on p. 242.

MERIDIAN ENERGIZING THERAPY

Anterior/Front

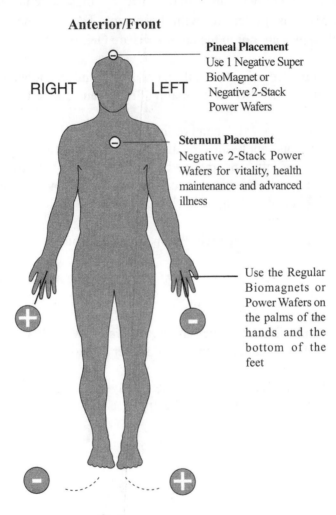

RIGHT   LEFT

Pineal Placement
Use 1 Negative Super
BioMagnet or
Negative 2-Stack
Power Wafers

Sternum Placement
Negative 2-Stack Power
Wafers for vitality, health
maintenance and advanced
illness

Use the Regular
Biomagnets or
Power Wafers on
the palms of the
hands and the
bottom of the
feet

⊖ These symbols indicate the polarity of
⊕ the Biomagnet that touches the skin.

BODY POLARITIES

OMET (Overnight MET) was developed for individuals whose protocols require multiple MET applications and who want to progress their therapy more quickly. They can do the MET while sleeping. Since the OMET is a much longer therapy than the standard MET, and to ensure that the energy is not too strong, the Power Wafer (PW) replaces the Regular Biomagnet (RB) in the therapy.

Following the standard MET polarity application, apply a single PW on each wrist above the hand, under each foot or on the back of the ankle, and the normal 2-Stack of PWs on the head. The OMET does not require the Daytime sternum placement. Apply the therapy as long as it feels good.

MET Nervousness experienced when first doing the MET indicates very low energy and toxic buildup. Do the Daytime or CVS therapy for 3-10 days to provide enough energy to detoxify, and then apply the MET comfortably with good results.

*Pacemaker/Defibrillator ♥PD WARNING, page 117.

Organ Group Energizing (OGE) Therapy: The OGE therapy is used for chronic illness or an injury that has led to a chronic medical condition. The OGE elevates and helps normalize the primary organ functions all at the same time (uniformly). This therapy helps overcome hypoactive, non-functioning organs to immediately normalize and start functioning properly. This also helps to re-start proper enzyme and hormone outputs in helping overcome chronic medical conditions and disease.

The OGE is so effective, it has helped awaken and heal a 91-year-old man out of a terminating septic shock coma (see *BioMagnificent Testimonials and Case Studies,* Chapter Thirteen). The OGE is often applied as the first therapy to re-start all the important metabolic functions. It is always applied in conjunction with other protocols such as the MET, Daytime, Nightime, etc., as shown in the ATACC (Acute Chronic Therapy Protocols) in the *Wellness Kit Pictorial Guide.*

However, it should be noted that many people use it 24/3 as a tune-up therapy for more energy.

OGE Placement: Using medical tape, band-aid or a bandage, apply four Negative 2-Stacks of PW/RB over:

- The liver under the forward right side of rib cage and the pancreas/ spleen under the forward left rib cage.
- Both Kidneys on the back – same level as the front placements.
- Place a Negative 2-Stack of PWs on CVS.

Term: 24 hours a day for 3-5 days depending upon the condition. The OGE therapy is available as a separate kit or in the Wellness Kit or separately, pgs. 188-190.

Organ Group Energizing Therapy

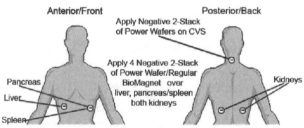

Please note that the 2-stack PW/RB Liver & Pancreas/Spleen
application energizes these primary organs uniformly

Brain Re-Entrainment Therapy (BRT): The BRT helps heal and normalize neurological dissociative and hypotrophic conditions, such as migraine headaches; infant manifest nystagmus with strabismus (blindness from lack of optokinetic development of the optic nerve, muscles and associative connective tissue); post-stroke motor functions; tremors; and depression. This is done by retraining and energizing the energy flow in the brain and increasing the energy in the neurotransmitter chemistry which helps signals clarify better.

The BRT is normally applied during the day along with the Daytime Therapy (♥PD WARNING*). *The CVS placement cannot be used during the BRT.*

BRT Application: During the day for 3-6 hours, apply a 2-Stack Negative PWs on the middle forehead on the skin with a band-aid at the hairline to stimulate the brain's energy to retrain its natural flow from the frontal lobe through the brain to the back of the head (occipital) and down into the body. The forehead placement can be left on all day and night unless other therapies (OMET, Nightime) are required.

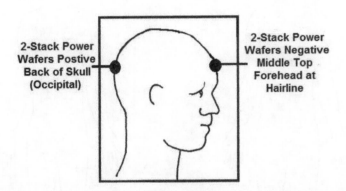

3-4 times during the BRT period, a 2-Stack Positive PWs is placed on the occipital (back of head/skull) for 10 minutes, then removed. The application provides a healing circuit of natural energy flow between the front Negative and back Positive placement to help correct any neurological issue.

*Pacemaker/Defibrillator ♥PD WARNING, page 117.

Body Polarities

The diagram of the body is shown in the "Anatomical View" with the thumbs out and palms facing front – an important understanding about the Polarity Meridians of the hands and arms.

The small dotted line that indicates the center division line between the Positive and Negative body polarities.

• • •PSL (Polarity Separation Line) • • •
PROPER POLARITY PLACEMENT (PPP)

BODY POLARITIES

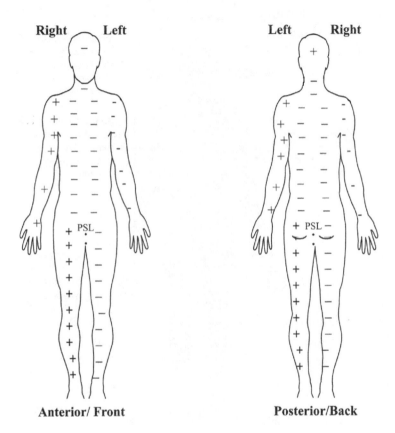

Anterior/ Front   Posterior/Back

PROPER POLARITY PLACEMENT (PPP)

Important Applications on Limbs

As noted in the Anatomical View (thumbs out, palm forward) in the
Polarity illustration on the previous page and the illustrations of the
body in the second part of this chapter, different parts of the body

have different charges. For Biomagnetic applications, the torso has a basically Negative charge. But the limbs (hands, feet, arms, legs, shoulder joints, and hips) are completely different. They have been measured and the charges are different from the left and right, front and back. On the limbs, each side is exactly the opposite charge of the other side. These areas are along what are called meridians.

The left anterior (front) meridian of the limbs has a Negative (-) polarity charge and the right anterior meridian of the limbs has a Positive (+) charge. Using the Anatomical View, we see that the left palm, wrist, arm, shoulder, hip, leg and top of the foot meridian have a Negative charge while the right palm, wrist, arm, shoulder, hip, leg and top of the foot meridian have the opposite Positive charge.

The posterior (back) of each side has exactly the opposite charge from its anterior (front) meridian. The posterior of the left limbs including the bottom of the foot has a Positive charge while the posterior of the right limbs including the bottom of the foot has a Negative charge.

Why the Polarity Meridians are so Important: When applying a strong magnetic field, such as with the Bio-Negative healing energy to the body, the magnetism excites the electrons and generates an electrical charge in the atoms that make up the cells. An electrical micro-current is also generated and flows from the point of application throughout the tissue.

The Biomagnetic energy is what increases the electrical energy and health of the cells and tissue while at the same time reducing pain.

Always Place Negative Energy on the Negative Meridian and Positive Energy on the Positive Meridian. *(See exception for skin and hip applications.)* Just as with your car or electronic device, the electrical energy in the body flows in a specific direction. If you have ever read the warning about using jumper cables on the battery of a car, the same warning applies to your body.

139

On the battery, you would never cross the Positive and Negative because it would spark dangerously, short circuit, and can cause major damage. On the limbs, applying Bio-Negative energy on a Positive Meridian or Bio-Positive energy on a Negative Meridian causes a short circuit in the body's energy flow and surrounding tissue. The improperly applied energy can prohibit healing and, as many people report, stress the area and cause pain.

Proper Polarity Placement (PPP): When the energy is applied correctly on the applicable meridian, the energy substantially enhances healing while providing rapid pain relief. The Proper Polarity Placement (PPP) refers to any therapy that is applied on the Meridians of the limbs and is shown on the body diagrams on the following pages and in the *Quick Reference Guide* on p. ix.

Application Placement: When using the PPP, review the Polarity diagram and note which side of your limbs is Positive and Negative. Then place the Bio-Negative Biomagnet on the Negative meridian even if the pain is in the Positive meridian on the other side of the limb. By applying the Bio-Negative energy on the Negative meridian, the healing energy naturally flows into the Positive Meridian to help quickly reduce pain and stimulate healing.

Example of Proper Polarity Placement (PPP)

Carpal Tunnel Example: Although the pain may be on the other side of the wrist, the PPP is applied as follows:

- If the pain is on the right wrist, apply the Negative green on the Posterior (opposite palm side) of the wrist. If the pain is on the left wrist, place the Negative green on the anterior (palm side) of the wrist.

- Wear for 3.5 days. If there is relief, continue wearing another 7 days to ensure enough healing time.

- However, if there is no relief after 3.5 days, apply the Circuit Therapy by applying the Positive on the anterior right wrist (palm side) or on the posterior left wrist (opposite palm side) along with the Negative BioMagnet and wear for 10 days.

- On the 11th day, remove the Positive and continue to wear the Negative for another 10 days to help complete the energy healing.

- If the pain returns after removing the Positive, re-apply the Positive to complete the Circuit Therapy for another 10 days.

- Then follow the same step by removing the Positive and continuing the Negative for another 10 days to help complete the healing.

Heel Example: If the problem area is the heel of the foot such as a fracture or trauma, placements of the biomagnets are as follows:

- On the right foot, place the Negative green on the bottom of the foot or back of the ankle on the Negative Meridian.

- On the left foot, place the Negative green on the top of the foot.

- Wear for 3.5 days. If there is relief, continue wearing another 7 days to ensure enough healing time.

- However, if there is no relief after 3.5 days, apply the Circuit Therapy by applying the Positive on the anterior right foot (top) or on the posterior left foot (bottom foot) along with the continuing Negative BioMagnet and wear for 10 days.

- On the 11th day, remove the Positive and continue to wear the Negative for another 10 days to help complete the energy healing.

- If the pain returns after removing the Positive, re-apply the Positive to complete the Circuit Therapy for another 10 days.

- Then follow the same step by removing the Positive and continuing the Negative for another 10 days to help complete the healing.

Right Foot   **Left Foot**

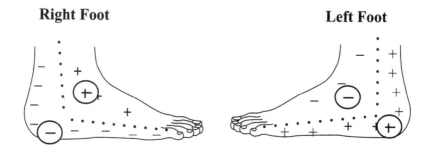

Proper Polarity Placement of the BioMagnet is very important on the shoulders, arms, legs extremities and on the hip when using Circuit Therapy.

BioMagnets are applied with band-aid, adhesive tape or self-stick bandage.

Examples of Rapid Meridian Healing

Example 1) A 72-year-old male crushed both knees and splintered both legs down to his ankles in an accident just before Thanksgiving. After operating and screwing everything together, his doctor explained it would take approximately ten months (till August) to heal, and then physiotherapy would be required for him to learn to walk again. After placing Super BioMagnets Bio-Negative green down in the Negative Meridians down the front of his left leg and back of his right, he needed no pain medicine and was walking normally by the third week of January – 400% faster healing without any complications or long-term physiotherapy.

Example 2) The following case required the Knee Circuit Therapy on the right leg to regenerate a severed nerve, which requires PPP. The nerve in the knee of a 72-year-old man was severed during surgery. His doctor said, "You will never feel anything below the knee ever again."

The man had reported to us that walking was extremely hard without having any feeling. We advised him to do the Knee Circuit therapy.

The Circuit therapy requires that on the right leg, the Bio-Positive be applied on the front of the leg below the knee in the Positive meridian and the Bio-Negative applied on the back of the leg above the knee in the Negative meridian.

After one month of the Knee Circuit Therapy, the nerve healed and he got his feeling back and could walk normally again. To see a video of him, go to www.BiomagScience.Net.

EXCEPTION to Proper Polarity Placement
Skin Conditions – Hip

Skin Condition – Negative Placement on a Positive Meridian: A single Power Wafer Bio-Negative green can be used on a Positive meridian for *20 Minutes ONLY for topical skin conditions* such as burns, cuts, insect bites, scrapes or baker's cysts. This will not interfere with the energy flow. Any longer *than a 20 minute application* is too strong and will short-circuit the natural energy flow and may cause pain.

HIP BONE Negative Placement on a Positive Meridian: The hip meridians are flexible and a powerful Bio-Negative energy may be used anywhere on either hip. However, if Circuit Therapy is required to help generate connective tissue, the PPP on the meridian is required.

Proper Polarity Placement Lateral View

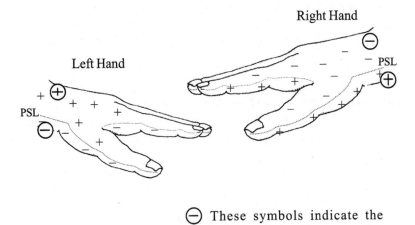

⊖ These symbols indicate the
⊕ polarity of the Biomagnet that
touches the skin

PSL – Polarity Separation Line • • • • •

Proper Polarity Placement Lateral View

Right

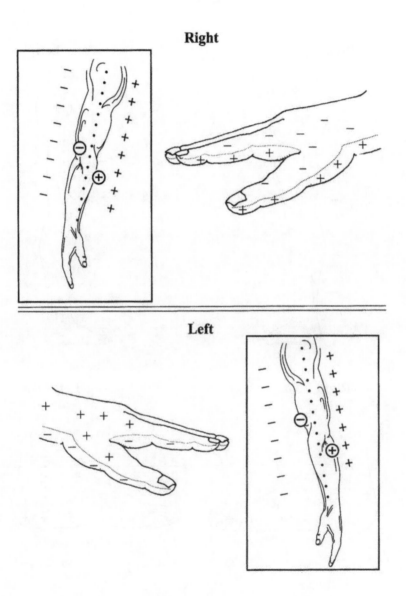

Left

Lateral View

Right   **Left**

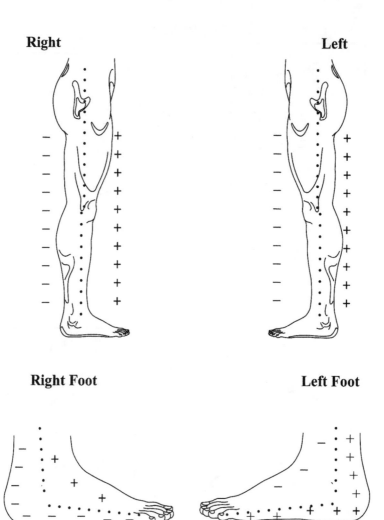

Right Foot   **Left Foot**

CIRCUIT THERAPY REGENERATION

Nerve, Fractures, Cartilage & Connective Tissue

Circuit Therapy ("CT"), formerly known as the Vortex Initiation Healing Therapy, helps heal and/or regenerate severed nerves, broken bones, and damaged, missing or worn-out cartilage and connective tissue by applying both the Bio-Negative and Bio-Positive fields in a circuit.

CT works like the body when a fracture occurs. The fracture first goes into a Positive and Negative charge on each side of the break to pull the bone together (opposite charges attract) to calcify and heal. Once the union is initiated, the site goes into a fully Negative charged state to heal.

In CT, the Bio-Negative and Bio-Positive energies are applied in the both the correct Negative and Positive Meridians (PPP-Proper Polarity Placement, p. 138) on both sides of the damaged or missing/severed soft tissue or fractured bone. Once the circuit is applied, the opposite energies are attracted to each other and reach out through the tissue to meet and balance with each other. Applications indicate that when there is any damaged or missing tissue in the middle of the Negative and Positive circuit that's preventing the flow of their energy from meeting, then their energy will stimulate the cells and their DNA to heal and/or regenerate the missing tissue so the energy can be bridged to meet and balance. Please see the miracle-like cases of severed nerves healed and quadriplegic walks again (Chapters Thirteen & Eighteen).

Circuit Therapy Protocols – Limbs, Shoulders, Hips, Back: Depending on the depth of penetration required, apply the appropriately sized BioMagnets (2-Stack: PWs, PW/RB or RBs) Bio-Negative and Bio-Positive 3 inches above and below (with the Negative application closest in the direction of the heart) or anterior (front) or posterior (back) on the site as required by the PPP, p. 138.

After 10 days, remove the Positive and place the Negative directly on the site for another 10 days to ensure healing. If pain occurs after removing the Positive, re-apply the Circuit (Positive) for another 10 days, then remove the Positive and apply the Negative over the site for 10 days.

Back, Sciatica, Herniated Discs: Apply a 2-Stack PWs Positive on spine and two 2-Stacks of PW/RB three inches to the right and left of the spine application. Wear for 10 days, then remove the spinal application and maintain the two left and right Negative placement for another 10 days. If pain returns after removing the center Positive, reapply the Positive spine application and repeat the protocol. Sciatica term: 3-4 weeks; Herniated discs term: 6-8 weeks.

See Circuit Therapy Applications in the *Wellness Kit Pictorial* Guide

IMPORTANT NOTE: It is important to do all BiomagScience therapies for the specified term to ensure the body has enough time to fully heal.

148

Proper Polarity Placement for
Fracture or Cartilage Repair

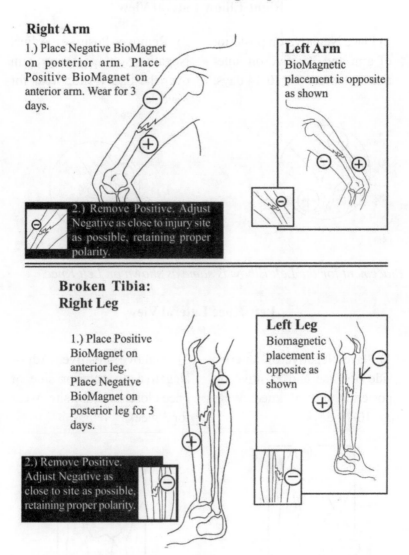

Right Arm
1.) Place Negative BioMagnet on posterior arm. Place Positive BioMagnet on anterior arm. Wear for 3 days.

2.) Remove Positive. Adjust Negative as close to injury site as possible, retaining proper polarity.

Left Arm
BioMagnetic placement is opposite as shown

Broken Tibia: Right Leg
1.) Place Positive BioMagnet on anterior leg. Place Negative BioMagnet on posterior leg for 3 days.

2.) Remove Positive. Adjust Negative as close to site as possible, retaining proper polarity.

Left Leg
Biomagnetic placement is opposite as shown

See "Fracture" in the Health Conditions and BioMagnetic Therapy Chapter.

Proper Polarity Placement for Fracture or Cartilage Repair

Right-Elbow Lateral View

1) Place Negative on posterior of arm and Positive on anterior arm. Wear for 10-14 days.

2) Remove Positive. Adjust Negative on posterior arm over the injury site. Wear for 3 weeks.

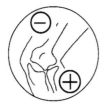

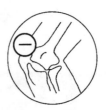

Placement for the Left Elbow is same as shown on Left Knee.

Left-Knee Lateral View

1) Place Negative on anterior side of knee and Positive on posterior side of knee. Wear for 10-14 days

2) Remove Positive. Adjust Negative on anterior side of knee close to injury site. Wear for 3 weeks

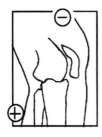

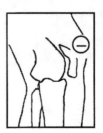

Placement for the right knee is same as shown on right elbow.

Nerve Regeneration

It has been shown that the electromagnetic forces from Biomagnetism can regenerate severed nerve cells. If the injury such as a broken neck, back, etc. just occurred, it is first important to reduce the inflammation at the trauma site or nerve breach. With your medical practitioner's approval, use the Circuit Therapy.

Spinal Regeneration Therapy Technique:

1. First apply Negative to the area for 3 days to reduce swelling/inflammation.
2. After the inflammation is reduced, apply a Negative 2-Stack of Power Wafers 2 inches above the nerve breach/break and a Positive 2-Stack of Power Wafers 2 inches below the breach/break. *No matter where the injury is, the Negative is always placed above the Positive toward the head.*
3. If the injury is old, start with Step 2 above. The therapy term may take months, but has shown results of new feeling, movement and eventual healing within a reasonable time.

Examples of Nerve Regeneration

After 20 doctors told him he would never walk again, a middle-aged man, almost completely quadriplegic, did the MET (Meridian Energizing Therapy) religiously and started to get feeling after a number of months. Working at it over a year, he got back full feeling, motion and normal use of his body. Unfortunately, the individual had not known that the spinal nerve regeneration protocol was available and may have been able to heal his spinal break much more quickly.

Another middle-aged male, quadriplegic for many years, got some feeling and motion back after the spinal nerve regeneration circuit was applied. Within a month of the application, the individual was able to raise his arm slowly and shake hands with our representative who had directed the therapy. Unfortunately, we lost contact with the man and do not have any follow-up. However, according to what we have learned and the fact that his spinal cord had already shown considerable healing, it is possible that he may have normalized.

After 6 months of physiotherapy, the doctor explained to a 72-year-old man whose nerve in his knee was severed during surgery, that he would never be able to feel anything from his knee down or ever have full motion of his leg again. (See video at BiomagScience.net.) Subsequently, the Knee Circuit Therapy was applied. In less than six weeks, his nerve and connective tissue regenerated for full feeling and motion and he was able to walk normally again.

BiomagScience Circuit Therapy Kits

Single Circuit Therapy kits such as for the back/sciatica, carpal, elbow, shoulder, hip, knee, Organ Group Energizing are available separately from BiomagScience. The Wellness Kit comes with all the magnets, material and instructions to encompass all the Circuit Therapies for whatever need may arise. The Wellness Kit is recommended as the most important, all-purpose First-Aid kit that everyone should have in their home for any emergency and for increasing and maintaining the family's vitality and good health.

CHAPTER NINETEEN

ILLUSTRATIONS

- **BioMagnetic Placement Location**
- **Overview of Body Organs and Glands**
- **Upper Body**
- **Digestive System**
- **Endocrine System**
- **Lymphatic System**
- **Urinary System**
- **Circulatory System**
- **Nervous System**

Illustrations

Overview of Body Organs and Glands
For BioMagnetic Placement Location

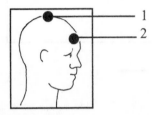

Lateral Head

Anterior Body

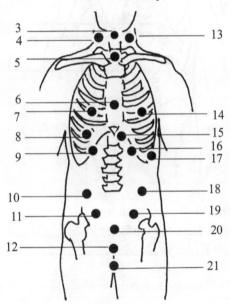

1. Pineal_____	8. Liver _____	16. Stomach_____
2. Pituitary_____	9. Gall bladder_____	17. Spleen _____
3. Thyroid_____	10. Ascending colon__	18. Descending colon_
4. Parathyroid_____	11. Right ovary_____	19. Left ovary_____
5. Thymus_____	12. Urinary bladder___	20. Uterus_____
6. Heart*_____	13. Parathyroid_____	21. Prostate_____
*Sternum placement	14. Lt. Lung_____	
7. Rt. Lung_____	15. Pancreas_____	

Name:

Date:

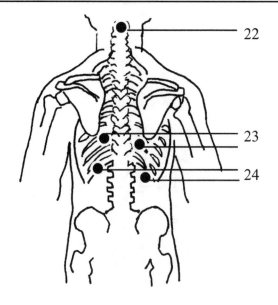

22. CVS (Cerebral Vestibular system)_____
23. Right and left Adrenals glands_____
24. Right and Left Kidneys_____

This chart is used for Magneto-Diagnostics and biomagnetic placement location.

Practitioner's note: Reaction to South Pole is Hyper Active
                         Reaction to North Pole is Hypo Active

Test • Record • Treat with opposite pole

Internal Organs of the Upper Body

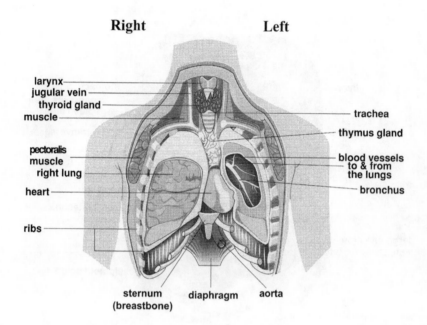

Right   Left

larynx
jugular vein
thyroid gland
muscle
trachea
thymus gland
pectoralis muscle
right lung
heart
blood vessels to & from the lungs
bronchus
ribs
sternum (breastbone)
diaphragm
aorta

Thyroid
Thymus
Pectoralis muscle
Heart
Lung – Bronchus
Diaphragm
Sternum (breastbone)

Sternum Placement is used for Daytime Therapy

Digestive System

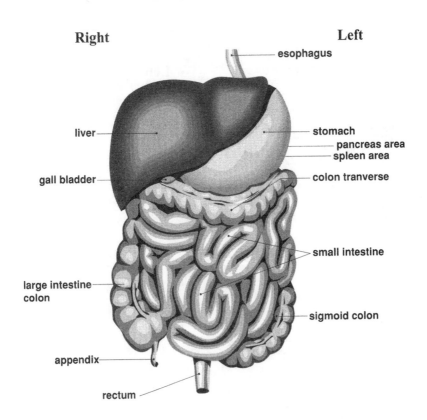

Right   Left

esophagus

liver   stomach
pancreas area
spleen area

gall bladder   colon tranverse

small intestine

large intestine
colon

sigmoid colon

appendix

rectum

Esophagus	**Large intestine (colon)**
Liver	**Tranverse colon**
Gall bladder	**Small Intestine**
Stomach	**Sigmoid colon**
Pancrea	**Appendix**
Spleen Rectum	

Endocrine System

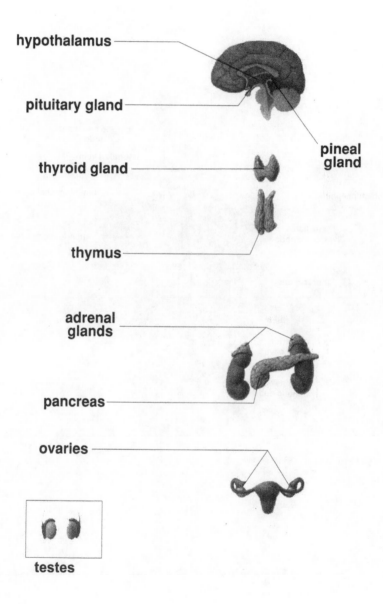

hypothalamus

pituitary gland

pineal
gland

thyroid gland

thymus

adrenal
glands

pancreas

ovaries

testes

Lymphatic System

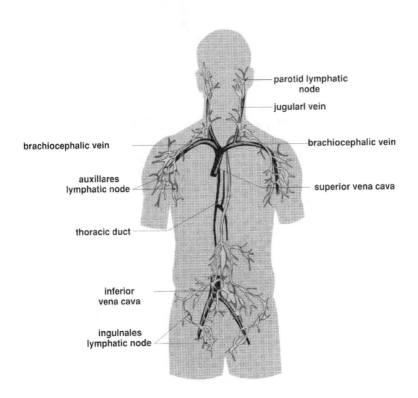

parotid lymphatic node

jugularl vein

brachiocephalic vein

brachiocephalic vein

auxillares lymphatic node

superior vena cava

thoracic duct

inferior vena cava

ingulnales lymphatic node

Urinary System

Right   Left

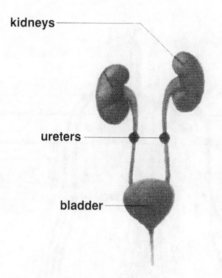

kidneys

ureters

bladder

Blood Circulation

Principal Veins and Arteries

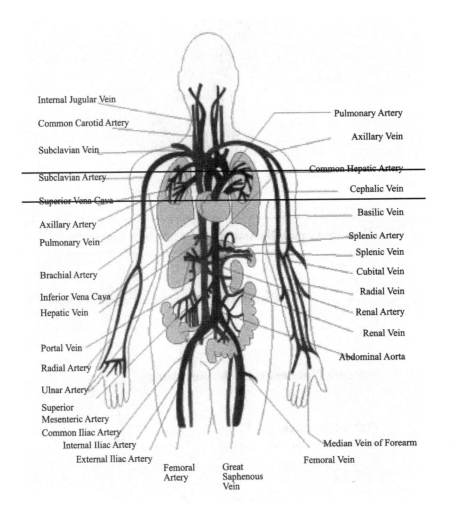

Internal Jugular Vein

Common Carotid Artery

Subclavian Vein

Subclavian Artery

Superior Vena Cava

Axillary Artery

Pulmonary Vein

Brachial Artery

Inferior Vena Cava

Hepatic Vein

Portal Vein

Radial Artery

Ulnar Artery

Superior
Mesenteric Artery

Common Iliac Artery

Internal Iliac Artery

External Iliac Artery

Femoral
Artery

Great
Saphenous
Vein

Pulmonary Artery

Axillary Vein

Common Hepatic Artery

Cephalic Vein

Basilic Vein

Splenic Artery

Splenic Vein

Cubital Vein

Radial Vein

Renal Artery

Renal Vein

Abdominal Aorta

Median Vein of Forearm

Femoral Vein

Nervous System

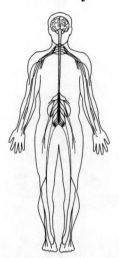

COMMONLY USED BIOMAGNETIC PLACEMENT LOCATIONS

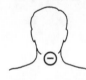 **CVS Placement:** On the back middle of the neck on the skin at the hairline.

Sternum Placement: On the breastbone, over the indentation of the sternum.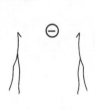

 Pineal Placement:
At the crown of the head

⊖ This symbol indicates the polarity of the Biomagnet that touches the skin.

CHAPTER TWENTY

CELLULAR RESEARCH

Prevention of Heart Attacks and Stroke

Hypercoagulation is a thickening of the blood where the RBCs (red blood cells) stack up and clump together in what is called the Rouleaux formation. It is one of the leading causes of heart attacks, strokes, high blood pressure and a host of other illnesses. (See the microscope pictures on the following pages.)

The stacking and clumping of RBCs reduces the RBC's surface area to the capillary beds, which reduces the delivery of oxygen (O^2) and nutrition to the tissue which also reduces the CO_2 exchange to the lungs. The reduced oxygen/nutrition and increased CO_2 results in cellular dysfunction, leading to conditions such as arthritis, atherosclerosis, autoimmune diseases, bone necrosis, cancer, cardiovascular diseases, chronic fatigue/CFS, chronic infections, deep vein thrombosis, dementia, depression, diabetes, eye diseases, fibromyalgia, heart attack, high blood pressure, infertility, Lyme disease, menstrual problems, metabolic syndrome (stuck cells), migraine, osteonecrosis of hips, knees and jaws, pulmonary embolism, stroke, tinnitus, and varicose veins.

Hypercoagulation also increases the blood's tendency to form fibrin (a sticky protein fiber) which can lead to excessive clotting in the blood, causing inflammation and creating obstruction in capillaries and the vascular system, leading to thrombosis and necrosis in tissue, veins, pulmonary embolism of the lungs, heart attack and stroke.

Thick Blood: Besides the clotting and fibrin, hypercoagulation thickens the blood viscosity which reduces the flow and increases blood pressure.

Blood thinners: Hypercoagulation creates a lot of medical problems and is why so many people use blood thinners like Coumadin (Warfarin), Pradaxa, Xarelto, Eliquis, just to list a few of the many that are available. Have you ever reviewed the safety information of blood thinners? They say, "…can cause bleeding, excessive bleeding, may lead to death"?

The possible side effects of blood thinners are scary. The fine print indicates once starting them, if you have to stop for surgery or dental work, the doctor should be notified, because stopping may cause a stroke or heart attack. In other words, taking blood thinners is precarious, but hypercoagulation is too dangerous not to do something about it. The following test shows how simple Biomagnetic therapy can help keep the blood thin naturally while providing even greater benefits.

The following microscope pictures of blood cell hyper-coagulation show how Biomagnetism thins the blood naturally while promoting increased health and wellness.

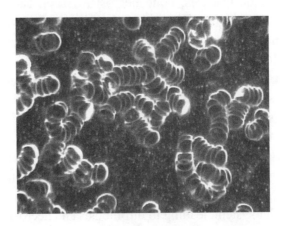

Hypercoagulation of Blood Cells

Sample 1: Live cell blood analysis of a 26-year-old male professional with a history of physical inactivity, poor nutrition, inadequate water consumption, difficulty sleeping and general malaise. He fasted the night before the test.

This RBC pattern of dehydration and inflammation is typical of many people with a poor diet who don't drink enough water and get very little exercise. The RBCs are stacking and clumping together (Rouleaux formulation) due to their loss of the Zeta potential which is the slight proper negative charge that is part of healthy RBCs which keeps them separated to provide normal nutritional/oxygen delivery and CO_2 detoxification from the tissue.

The small floating specks are a large amount of fats probably from the individual's fast food diet. Normally fats are cleared from the blood within four hours of ingestion, however hydrogenated fats have been observed to take days; in this case, it may take quite awhile to clear from the blood, even with an immediate diet change.

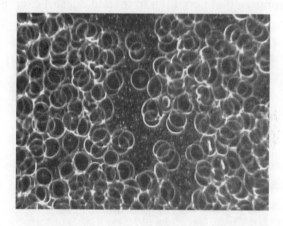

Sample 2: After 30 minutes of BiomagScience Therapy

Sample 2: Observed after 30 minutes of BiomagScience Sternum Therapy, this shows improvement in plasma congestion and a partial improvement in the Rouleaux formulation as well as the fats (specks).

The smallest size fats are HDL's, medium sizes are LDL's, and the very large fats may be cylomicrons or hydrogenated fats from a fast food diet. Fats enter the body in the microvilli (finger-like projections in the small intestine that emulsify the ingested fats) into the lacteal duct (the lymphatic system). This is very significant due to the fact that the lymphatic system houses our immune system and powerful antioxidants that the liver creates.

The fats are then dumped into the subclavian vein and into the blood stream. One can only imagine the congestion this can cause with a constant diet high in harmful fats including hydrogenated and partially hydrogenated oils.

Another important issue is that the lymphatic system does not have a pump like the arterial system does. Some of the ways it is able to circulate include exercise, through the pumping action of the muscles, and deep breathing which changes the thoracic pressure to create movement both in the lymphatic system as well as the venous System. This is significant in this case due to the fact that this individual consumes a diet very high in fat and doesn't exercise.

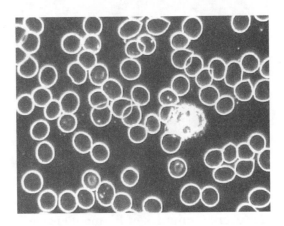

Sample 3: After 2.5 hours of BiomagScience Sternum Therapy

Sample 3: After 2.5 hours of BiomagScience Sternum Therapy, the Zeta Potential was reinstated in the RBCs, which separated and normalized, significantly improving circulation. The sample also shows the White Blood Cells (WBC's) with increased motility and since the fats have been cleared, verifies the Bio-Negative Energy Therapy has supported a substantial increase in liver and gallbladder functions. The blood chemistry is now normal.

After the BiomagScience Energy Therapy, the unhealthy and dangerous effects of hypercoagulation of the blood chemistry was resolved. The low [Zeta potential] energy of the RBCs that creates the thick blood viscosity responsible for so many health problems including heart attack and stroke was resolved by the Bio-Negative energy therapy in just 2.5 hours. Furthermore, the Bio-Negative energy also increased the RBCs motility (metabolic functions) which was conveyed to increased organ and lymphatic functions.

Conclusion: Biomagnetic energy therapy is a natural method to quickly thin the blood and eliminate hypercoagulation while positively increasing nutrition, detoxification and other important metabolic functions in the body without any bad side effects. The therapy also supports preventive maintenance for good health – something that drug thinners cannot provide. The BiomagScience OGE, MET, and CVS therapies provide the same energy support to overcome hypercoagulation of the blood.

*Note: Bio-Energized Structured water was not taken during the test. It has been shown that when used in conjunction with the BiomagScience therapy, the charged structured water works synergistically in providing further support in nutrition/oxygen delivery and detoxification of the cells.

Dry-Cell Oxidative Stress test of Free-Radical sites
Taken concurrently with RBC tests above

The following is the effect on the free-radicals BiomagScience therapy had on the 26-year-old. Take a look at the following before and after microscope pictures of the free-radical sites:

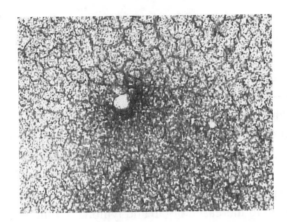

Sample 1 – Dry, Untreated – Taken Prior to Energy Therapy: The dry cell Bowen Test shows evidence of oxidative stress/free radical activity that is observed in this sample as the white round cell near the center. This is the indicator of free radical activity in all the tissue.

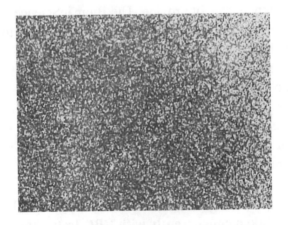

Sample 2.5 hours after Energy Therapy

The dry cell has filled in and healed in the matter of 2.5 hours, showing no free radical activity. "In my many years of clinical experience, I have never before seen this kind of dramatic change."

~ C. B. (BiomagScience Researcher)

Conclusion of BiomagScience Therapy on Free Radicals Site

The Bio-Negative Energy of BiomagScience therapy produces an abundance of Negative electromotive healing energy which, like the donor electrons of anti-oxidants, neutralizes the positively charged free-radicals and provides supportive healing to the sites damaged by them. As observed by the researcher, the Biomagnetic therapy produced immediate rapid healing never seen before.

General Therapy Recommendations to Maintain
Wellness & Longevity

Using the Daytime therapy of a 2-Stack of BiomagScience PWs or RBs (Power Wafers or Regular BioMagnets), Bio-Negative is placed Green against the skin over the primary energizing point, the sternum (the heart) daily. Placement for men: inside and outside of the shirt; women: on the bra front strap or inside and outside inside the left cup next to the front strap.

Detoxification of the cells and the system is very important to good health. It is an immediate and natural response to Bio-Negative energy therapy.

If the individual indicates they feel a bit nervous or nauseous when first doing the sternum heart therapy, it is because they have very low energy and have built up a lot of toxins in their system. When the cells start to charge, they start to dump all the toxins, which can nervousness or nausea. If this occurs, simply reduce the power of the therapy by removing the 2-Stack of PWs and place them Green on the lower CVS – middle back of the neck on the skin at the hairline.

The lower CVS therapy will naturally thin the blood in about a day and will comfortably slow down the detoxification; the lower CVS can be applied all day for about 3-10 days before re-applying the Daytime (sternum) therapy on a daily basis. It is a personal choice.

Cellular Electrical Analysis with BIA Testing

The Bioelectrical Impedance Analysis (BIA) machine is an FDA registered instrument that analyzes and measures the electrical values of the cells, the parallel capacitance of the membrane and the voltage of the cytoplasm. The properties of the BIA circuit in the body are well defined. The method of measurement is precise, and sensitive in its ability to illustrate specific changes inherent in the subject.

The BIA provides a scientific index, a "snapshot" of cellular level dynamics and architecture, giving valuable and immediate data on the individual's state of health and before and after data from many protocols, including medical research, health care analysis and clinical practice recommendation.

BIA prediction measurement equations have been developed since 1939. The measurements use cellular membrane parallel resistance and reactance as predictors of intracellular, extracellular and body cell mass. These equations can specify if cellular health is static, progressing or regressing and have been an excellent tool in analyzing the efficacy of Biomagnetic therapies.

The BIA measurements show how effective and how quickly BiomagScience advanced therapies have helped individuals with acute and long-term chronic conditions start healing immediately. The results have been amazing.

Parallel Capacitance

All living things are made of cells and their membranes are bound compartments filled with a concentrated solution of chemicals, nutrients, elements, and salts. Groups of cells perform specialized functions and are linked by an intricate communications system.

The cell membrane maintains an ion concentration 'gradient' between the intracellular (internal cell/cytoplasm) and extracellular (external) environment. This electromotive difference between the surface of the inner and outer membrane is measured in pF (pico

Farads) and is known as the Parallel Capacitance. This difference is essential for efficient transfer of oxygen, nutrition, waste, and carbon dioxide in and out of the cell. The higher the capacitance, the healthier the cell is.

The Parallel Capacitance is not affected by weight or body fat. It is a measure of cellular health and changes dramatically, depending upon one's health. As unhealthy cells take on nourishment, their vitality and their parallel capacitance increases as they progress toward health. Inversely, as cells lose their energy and vitality, their capacitance goes down.

A very healthy person has a high [cellular] parallel capacitance whereas a malnourished or ill individual has a low parallel capacitance.

Increasing Capacitance

Any protocols and/or supplements that progress the body's health will show an increased capacitance. Inversely, any substances that decrease the capacitance need further inspection.

The BIA instrument provides data points. The more data points the greater ability to make an accurate diagnosis that can best assist the client. For example, someone detoxifying or going through a life change can ultimately experience a major shift in health and capacitance. There are some exceptions such as an immediate detoxification that will lower capacitance before a breakthrough [shift] will raise it.

Normally it takes as many as 6 months of strict diet and lifestyle change to increase the parallel capacitance more than 50 pF. However, within an hour of Biomagnetic therapy, the pF was increased over 100pF. This had never been seen before.

Parallel capacitance cellular health table for females

Capacitance	Cell health based on parallel capaticance
(pF - pico Farads)	Extremely healthy
Above 1009	Optimal health
774-1008	Average
617-773	Below average
460-616	Low energy
304-459	Warning alert
Below 303	

Parallel capacitance cellular health table for males

Capacitance	Cell health based on parallel capacitance
(pF - pico Farads)	Extremely healthy
Above 1313	Optimal health
1003-1312	Average
795-1002	Below average
589-794	Low energy
382-588	Warning alert
Below 381	

The following BIA test shows the before and after cellular voltage and health using BiomagScience therapy protocols

BIA – Parallel Capacitance Body Composition
Report # 111804MW

History: The subject, a 53-year-old female, had a history of malabsorption, fibromyalgia, and extreme fatigue that incapacitated her and kept her bedridden for 25 years. Malabsorption is when the cell has so little voltage, it cannot pull in the necessary micro-nutrients to increase its energy – a very bad Catch 22 situation. She has been under the care of a multitude of practitioners who have not been able to help her. She even tried using very weak, improperly designed magnets. She tests for chemical poisoning. Due to her malabsorption issues, she cannot take any supplements; even a slight nutritional supplementation created an overload and throws her body into a crisis.

During the last three years prior to the BiomagScience therapy, her capacitance was very low, only rising 25 points after multiple therapies, including a custom nutritional program. The subject's inability to absorb or detoxify made it very difficult for her health to improve and most therapies made her ill.

Parallel capacitance results of Subject 111804MW

Date	18-Nov-04	14-Jun-05	14-Jun-05
Actual CAP:	400	400	507

Note: From Nov 4th to June 5th the subject's capacitance remained the same even with a diet high in nutrition, but minimal supplementation, due to malabsorption, which was typical of her fixed pattern. After her BIA test and within an hour of using the CVS application, her cellular capacitance rose 107 points, indicating a large increase in the cell's voltage and health progression.

Description	Actual	Norm	Diff	Normal Range	Comment
18-Nov-04	400	706	-305	Min: 558 Max: 855 (PF)	CAP less than min by 158.0 (pico farads)
14-Jun-05	400	706	-305	Min: 558 Max: 855 (PF)	CAP less than min by 158.0 (pico farads)
14-Jun-05	507	706	-199	Min: 558 Max: 855 (PF)	CAP less than min by 51.0 (pico farads)

After the CVS therapy, within a month of Bio-Negative energized water and BiomagScience Daytime, Nightime, and MET therapies, the subject was able to get her life back and resume her favorite activity of singing and song-writing with a band.

This dynamic improvement was monumental, as the subject had been unable to perform the most basic activity for 25 years, including standing for any periods without severe pain. The chemical poisoning that she suffered from resulted in blocking important pathways, reducing her energy so low that she did not have the electromotive energy in her cells for complete metabolic function.

Her cell's chronically stuck, low-charged voltage was immediately elevated by the BiomagScience therapy to a properly charged functioning state. This re-started the cells' natural ionic forces to be able to metabolize micronutrients, resulting in increased metabolic and immune functions, which started her back on the road to full recovery. Her state of health had been stuck in a toxic pattern for 25 years that nothing helped, until she applied BiomagScience energy therapies. Within a year of the BiomagScience initial therapy, she was playing competitive tennis.

Conclusion

The BIA test shows and verifies BiomagScience proper energy therapy supplementation immediately elevates the cellular energy and immune functions for overcoming critical health issues heretofore not able to be resolved. This case indicates just a minor segment of health issues not treatable with allopathic medicine: cases that now have scientific energy therapies and protocols that help the body to quickly overcome pain and start of the road to healing.

BiomagScience's specific therapies also provide the necessary energy to stimulate the DNA to regenerate nerve and soft and hard tissue back to normal; this is shown in such cases as a paraplegic almost fully quadriplegic walking again or how herniated discs grew back to full height or separated nerves regenerated.

See additional BIA before and after testing on BiomagScience's web site: www.BiomagScience.net

CHAPTER TWENTY ONE

HEALTH CONDITIONS AND BIOMAGSCIENCE THERAPIES

General Therapy Review

Before starting any of the therapies, it is important to read a few of the chapters of basic therapy requirements and the simple precautions that should be followed to ensure the best results and to make sure the therapy is applied correctly so no stress is occurring to the body.

Pease read and familiarize yourself with the following:

1. Bio-Magnetic Precautions, Chapter 15.
2. Basics – How to use BioMagnetics, Chapter 17.
3. Products, Chapter 17.
4. Basic Biomagnetic Therapy Techniques, Chapter 18.
5. Proper Polarity Placement, Chapter 18 if you are applying it on any part of a limb.
6. Illustrations, Chapter 19.
7. Review the following abbreviations so you can understand the therapy.

Important: Please be aware of the ♥PD WARNING notice. Pacemaker Defibrillator WARNING: Do not place a magnet within 8" of the heart, p. 117.

If you have any questions, contact BiomagScience by phone, email or the forum at MagneticTherapyToday@YahooGroups.com.

Abbreviations used in Therapies

BioMagnet Configurations and Polarity Field:
- **PW**: Power Wafer • **RB**: Regular • **Super**: Super BioMagnet
- **2-Stack PW**: 2 Power Wafers stacked together
- **2-Stack RB**: 2 Regular Biomagnets stacked together
- **2-Stack PW/RB**: Power Wafer & Regular Biomagnet stacked together
- **Neg**: Bio-Negative Energy Field
- **Pos**: Bio-Positive Energy Field
- **PPP**: Proper Polarity Placement

Biomagnetic therapies:
- **ATACC**: The full Advanced Therapies for Acute/Chronic Conditions are in the *Wellness Kit Pictorial Guide**
- **BRT:** Brain Re-Entrainment Therapy, p. 136
- **CT**: Circuit Therapy (Vortex Healing), p. 147
- **CVS**: Lower Cerebellar Vestibular System, 2-Stack PWs Neg middle back of neck on skin at hairline, p. 163, 171, 229
- **Daytime**: Neg 2-Stack PWs over Sternum all day, p.130, 157
- **MET:** Meridian Energizing Therapy, p. 131
- **Nightime**: Top of head Neg 2-Stack PWs, p. 131
- **OGE**: Organ Group Energizing therapy, p. 135

*Note: The ATACC therapy protocols are only in the *Wellness Kit Pictorial Guide*. The entire Wellness Kit is required in order to perform all the therapies in the ATACC protocols.

Supplements required or recommended in the therapies:

- **BAO**: BiomagScience Activated Oxygen, normal dosage, p. 53
- **BNW:** Drink Bio-Negative Energized Structured water, p. 41
- **CE**: Circulation Enzymes Oral Chelation, normal 3-month term, p. 125, 247

- **hGH**: Ultimate Supplement Bio-Identical hGH, 6-12 months, p. 125, 247
- **Nutrition**: See Chapter 9 for Nutritional Support.
- **Nutritionist**: Important to consult with Medical Nutritionist.

A-Z HEALTH CONDITIONS

BIOMAGSCIENCE THERAPIES

Acne: Neg 2-Stack PW applied for 30 minutes minimum daily on area of outbreak. Wash area with 1/4th cup BNW and 50 drops BAO. Drink BNW with normal dosage BAO. Daytime (♥PD WARNING), Nightime for 2 weeks. See Nutrition. Eliminate sugar, fried and fatty foods. Term: 2-6 weeks.

Addictive States: Food, chemical or drugs. Drink BNW, Daytime (♥PD WARNING), CVS minimum 5-6 hours daily 2 months; Nightime important, Nutrition, Vitamin C IV for heroin addiction to eliminate DTs. Term: 3-16 weeks.

Alcoholism-related conditions: OGE 24/3, Neg Super on liver, diaphragm and pancreas for 10 minutes daily. Daytime (♥PD WARNING), Nightime, drink 4-6 glasses of BNW, see Nutrition. Term: 1-4 months.

Allergic Reactions:
Eye Reactions: Neg Single PW over each eye on mask all night. Rinse with BNW and drinking dose of BAO. Daytime, (♥PD WARNING), Nightime, CVS 24/7 for 2 weeks, Nutrition, Nutritionist, Vitamin A essential.

Abbreviations, p. 178, How to use BioMagnets, p. 123, Illustrations, p. 153, Energized Structured Water, p. 41, BAO Dosage, p. 53, ♥PD WARNING Sign (Pacemaker/Defibrillator WARNING) p. 117, Therapies p.129.

Gastrointestinal Reaction: MET for 30-45 minutes 3 times daily for 3 days, then once a day for 2 weeks. Neg Super BioMagnet for 2-3 hours on the stomach for calming effect. If gastric pain continues, use Pos Super BioMagnet for 10 minutes. Then repeat Neg procedure. Drink BNW with BAO. Supplement with Probiotic (at health food stores) to renew necessary colonic bacteria. (♥PD WARNING)

Amenorrhoea: Scanty or no menses. Daytime (♥PD WARNING), Nightime, drink BNW with BAO, optional ATACC. See Nutrition, Multivitamin/Mineral supplement, Nutritionist.

Ankles (Swollen): Apply the ATACC in *Wellness Kit Pictorial Guide*. In addition, continue with 2-Stack PW/RB on both kidneys 3-5 hours a day for 10 days after OGE. Use CE therapy for 3 months (♥PD WARNING), Nutrition.

Anxiety: Daytime (♥PD WARNING), Nightime, CVS 24/7 for 2 months, drink BNW, Nutrition. Calcium, magnesium and B-vitamins.

Appendicitis: See a physician immediately. Neg Super over appendix.

Arteriosclerosis and Atherosclerosis: Hardening of the arteries. Apply the ATACC in the *Wellness Kit Pictorial Guide* (♥PD WARNING). Supplement CE for 3 months chelation & cholestene 6 months, Nutrition, Term: 3 months.

Daily Supplementation: Taurine to remove fat – 500 mg., 2-3 times daily. Taurine is the building block of all the amino acids. A key component for the digestion of fats, it also controls serum cholesterol and the absorption of fat-soluble vitamins and is vital for the proper utilization of sodium, potassium, calcium and magnesium. BiomagScience CE oral chelation supplement reduces vascular and cellular plaque. It is suggested that L-arginine be supplemented to soften arteries and veins along with cholestene to reduce triglycerides and LDL.

Arthritis: Apply the ATACC in the *Wellness Kit Pictorial Guide*. Follow with Daytime (♥PD WARNING), Nightime, MET once a day for 2 weeks after ATACC and drink BNW with BAO. For specific areas of the limbs, check PPP for correct Neg placement, p. 138. Therapy terms: several months although major relief has been shown to occur within 7-10days. For chronic arthritis, follow the protocols above and tape the Neg PWs on the Neg meridian (PPP) as follows:

- feet and hands for 10 days;
- next, wrists and ankles for 10 days,
- then knees and elbows for 10 days,
- next, shoulders and hips for 10 days.

Continue the Daytime and drink BNW to maintain high energy defense against arthritis.

Asthma: Super or 2-Stack RBs Neg for 4-6 hours on both lungs daily for 2-3 weeks. MET 30-45 minutes daily for 2 months, Daytime (♥PD WARNING), Nightime, drink BNW with BAO. Consult physician, 2-3 grams liposomal vitamin C daily.

Asthma with acute bronchospasm: Super or 2-Stack RBs Neg for 4-6 hours on both lungs. Daytime (♥PD WARNING), Nightime, drink 4 glasses of BNW and with BAO in 2 glasses daily. Suggested to cut down and/or eliminate milk and milk products. Nutrition. See allergist for testing.

Athlete's Foot: See Infection, External.

Abbreviations, p. 178, How to use BioMagnets, p. 123, Illustrations, p. 153, Energized Structured Water, p. 41, BAO Dosage, p. 53, ♥PD WARNING Sign (Pacemaker/Defibrillator WARNING) p. 117, Therapies p.129.

Attention Deficit Disorder: CVS 24/7 for 2-3 months. Daytime (♥PD WARNING), Nightime; drink 4 glasses of BNW with BAO in 2 glasses daily. Nutrition, Nutritionist.

Backache/Sciatica: Back Circuit Therapy: For 10 days, use Pos 2-Stack PWs on the spine where pain is located. Place two Neg 2-Stacks PW/RB 3 inches on both sides of the Pos spine application. After ten days, remove the center Pos application and continue wearing the right and left Neg PW/RBs for 2 weeks. If pain returns after removing the center Pos, replace the Pos for another 10 days and then remove and continue wearing the right and left Neg applications for another 2 weeks. Daytime (♥PD WARNING), Nightime, drink BNW, Nutrition. Term: 3-8 weeks.

Baldness and Graying Hair: OGE 24/3, MET 30-45 minutes daily for 2 months. Daytime (♥PD WARNING), CVS daily, Nightime, drink BNW, hGH supplementation for 6-12 months. See Nutrition.

Bites (Insects, Bees): Neg R immediately on location for 2 hours to neutralize toxicity of sting and pain. Wash with BNW and BAO. Term: 2-4 hours.

Bites (Dog Bite): Neg Super on location. Wash with BNW and BAO. Contact physician immediately.

Bladder and Kidney: Apply the ATACC in the *Wellness Kit Pictorial Guide* along with 2-Stack Neg PW/RB over bladder and kidney(s) for 2 weeks, drink BNW with BAO, Diet: cabbage and wheat juice flush, 2-3 grams liposomal Vitamin C daily, Nutrition, Nutritionist. Term: 5 days to 2-3 weeks.

Blood Pressure – High Blood Pressure: Apply the ATACC in the *Wellness Kit Pictorial Guide*, follow with Daytime (♥PD WARNING), CVS daily, Nightime, drink 4 glasses BNW daily with BAO in 2 glasses, supplement 3 month CE and 6-12 month hGH. Consult your physician. Term: 3-4 months.

Bone Spurs of the Foot: Negative 2-Stack PWs on upper or lower foot (ankle or heel) PPP, p. 138. Possible Circuit therapy required, see *Wellness Kit Pictorial Guide*. Daytime (♥PD WARNING), Nightime, Nutritionist for supplementation. Term: 2-6 weeks.

Breast Lumps: Fibrocystic Breast: Use Neg Super or 2-Stack RBs over lump 24/7, minimally all day. Daytime (♥PD WARNING), CVS, Nightime, supplement 2-3 grams liposomal vitamin C daily, Nutrition, reduce red meat, carbohydrates, sugar, and increase vegetables, Nutritionist, drink 4 glasses BNW daily with BAO in 2 glasses. Term: 2-6 weeks.

Broken Bones: See Fractures, p. 149.

Bronchitis: Neg Super or 2-Stack RBs on left and right lungs 24/2, (♥PD WARNING) then OGE 24/3, then reapply Neg Super or 2-Stack RBs on left and right lungs 24/7 until resolution. MET 45 minutes x 2 daily for 5 days morning, afternoon after OGE, Nightime. Vitamins E, D and 2-3 grams daily liposomal vitamin C. Antibiotics may be necessary, consult physician, supplement professional probiotic to replace colonic bacteria killed by antibiotics. Term: Until condition is relieved.

Abbreviations, p. 178, How to use BioMagnets, p. 123, Illustrations, p. 153, Energized Structured Water, p. 41, BAO Dosage, p. 53, ♥PD WARNING Sign (Pacemaker/Defibrillator WARNING) p. 117, Therapies p.129.

183

Burns: Immediately wash and spray with 1/4th cup BNW with 50 drops BAO. If burn is 2nd degree, continue to spray with BNW/BAO mixture. If the area is a small burn, spray with mixture and place a single or 2-stack PWs Neg over burn for rapid healing, drink BNW with BAO and drink Bio-Energized Gatorade/electrolyte type of drink to support healing, supplement electrolytes and additional vitamins/minerals. Drink and spray constantly until healed. Daytime (♥PD WARNING), Nightime. 2-3 grams liposomal vitamin C daily. Term: 10-14 days for 2nd degree, 3-4 weeks for 3rd degree. Energized Structured Water, p. 41, BAO Dosage p. 53, ♥PD WARNING.

Bursitis: Depending upon location need, Neg 2-Stack PWs or PW/RBs on PPP (p. 138) over location. If no comfort is achieved in 3 days, then apply Circuit Therapy on location. Drink 4 glasses BNW daily with BAO in 2 glasses, consult Nutritionist. Daytime (♥PD WARNING), CVS, Nightime. Term: 3-6 weeks.

Calcium Deposits: See Arthritis, above. Apply the ATACC in the *Wellness Kit Pictorial Guide*, then follow up with MET 30-45 minutes once a day for 2 months, Daytime (♥PD WARNING), Nightime, see Nutrition, consult Nutritionist. Term: 2-3 months.

Cancer:

1. Neg Super over any tumor location(s) for 24/7.

2. Neg Super Daytime (♥PD WARNING) 24/7. If ♥PD, then 2-stack RB over CVS 24/7 except during bathing.

3. CVS daily.

4. Nightime for increased melatonin values.

5. Supplement 5-6 grams liposomal vitamin C daily; small build, 5 grams; medium to large build, 6 grams.

6. Drink 4-6 glasses BNW daily with BAO in 2 glasses.

Diet change essential. Reduce and/or eliminate red meat, carbohy-drates, sugar [products] and increase vegetables for alkaline diet. See Nutrition, consult Nutritionist. Term: 6-8weeks, continue with Daytime (♥PD WARNING), Nightime, reduce Vitamin C to 2-3 grams daily. Drink BNW.

Carotid Arteries: Apply ATACC in the *Wellness Kit Pictorial Guide* & apply Neg 2-Stack PWs on each artery 24/7 – take off if uncom-fortable, but re-apply thereafter minimally 2-3 hours a day. Important: 3 month CE supplementation, following ATACC: Daytime (♥PD WARNING), Nightime, drink 4 glasses BNW with BAO in two glasses daily. See Arteriosclerosis, above. Term: 2-3 months.

Carpal Tunnel: Neg 2-Stack PW on PPP on wrist for pain. Term: 10 days. If after 3.5 days there is no relief, then apply Negative/Positive Circuit Therapy for 10 days, then remove Pos and apply Neg for another 10 days.

Cartilage Regeneration: Joint, hip, shoulder, etc. See Circuit Therapy in the *Wellness Kit Pictorial Guide*; apply Neg/Pos CT in PPP for 4-8 weeks depending upon severity, then remove Pos and reapply Neg directly over the site for another 2 weeks. If the pain returns after removing the Pos, reapply the Pos for another 2 weeks, then remove and place Neg over site for 2 weeks to ensure healing time. Recommended CMO (Cetyl Myristoleate: health food store, on-line) supplementation for connective tissue regeneration, double daily dosage during the therapy term. Daytime (♥PD WARNING), Nightime, drink BNW with BAO. Term: Approx. 4-6 weeks.

Abbreviations, p. 178, How to use BioMagnets, p. 123, Illustrations, p. 153, Energized Structured Water, p. 41, BAO Dosage, p. 53, ♥PD WARNING Sign (Pacemaker/Defibrillator WARNING) p. 117, Therapies p.129.

Cataracts: One Neg PW on temple at end of eye socket 24/7 until relief. CVS 24/7 to vasodilate brain blood barrier to increase circulation, important to drink 4 glasses BNW with BAO in two glasses daily, 3 month CE supplementation to reduce plaque and increase circulation, Daytime (♥PD WARNING), Nightime. Consult Nutritionist for specialized eye supplementation. Term: 2-6 weeks.

Cellulite Deposits: Neg 2-Stack PWs or PW/RB worn on fatty tissue. Daytime (♥PD WARNING), Nightime, drink BNW with BAO. See Nutrition. Eliminate carbohydrates and all sugar for 6 weeks, reduce red meat and increase vegetables, exercise important. Term: 3-6 months.

Chemical Exposure: If hypersensitive, use Neg 2-Stack PWs on CVS 30 minutes the first day, then increase 15 minutes each day thereafter until 4 hour application (15 days), then apply the ATACC in the *Wellness Kit Pictorial Guide* (♥PD WARNING), follow with Super or 2-stack RBs Neg on liver and spleen daily for minimum 3-4 hours for 2 weeks. Drink 4-6 glasses of BNW with BAO in 2 glasses daily. Important CE chelation supplement 2-3 months, 2 grams daily of liposomal Vitamin C, and green algae or Spirulina. Term: 2-4 weeks.

Childhood Diseases: Daytime (♥PD WARNING), Nightime. Drink 4 glasses BNW with BAO in 2 glasses. See Nutrition. Term: normal.

Cholesterol and Triglycerides: See Arteriosclerosis, above. MET 45 minutes in the morning, Daytime (♥PD WARNING), Nightime. Drink 4 glasses BNW with BAO in two glasses daily. Important: CE chelation for 3 months, hGH and cholestene supplementation for 6-12 months. See Nutrition. Term: 2-6 months.

Chronic Fatigue Syndrome – CFS, includes Fibromyalgia, Candidiasis: If hypersensitive to supplements indicating malabsorption, use Negative 2-Stack PWs on CVS 30 minutes the first day, then increase 15 minutes each day thereafter until 4 hour application (15 days) is achieved, then apply the ATACC in the *Wellness Kit Pictorial Guide*, follow with continuous Daytime (♥PD WARNING), CVS minimum all day, Nightime, Drink 4 glasses BNW with BAO in two glasses daily, supplement hGH 6-12 months, 2-3 grams liposomal vitamin C daily. See Nutrition, consult Nutritionist. Term: 4-10 weeks.

Circulation: (poor) from diabetes, post-polio syndrome, Reynaud's, arteriosclerosis, etc. See Arteriosclerosis, above. 2-6 months.

Cirrhosis – Liver: Apply the ATACC in the *Wellness Kit Pictorial Guide* and Neg Super or 2-Stack RBs over liver all day for 1 month, then 4 hours daily for 2 more weeks. Continue with Daytime (♥PD WARNING), CVS daily for 2 week minimum, Nightime for 1 month, MET twice a week for 45 minutes. Drink 4 glasses BNW with BAO in two glasses daily, reduce alcohol consumption. See Nutrition, Chapter 9 for correct supplementation. Term: 4-6 weeks.

Colds: Daytime 2-Stack RB (♥PD WARNING), Nightime and CVS 24/14 to help clear sinuses. Drink 4 glasses BNW with 2 glasses BAO daily. Vitamin C: 3 grams immediately and 2 grams every 4 hour during 1st day, then 3 grams daily to relieve symptoms. See Nutrition.

Abbreviations, p. 178, How to use BioMagnets, p. 123, Illustrations, p. 153, Energized Structured Water, p. 41, BAO Dosage, p. 53, ♥PD WARNING Sign (Pacemaker/Defibrillator WARNING) p. 117, Therapies p.129.

Colitis: Apply the ATACC in Pictorial Guide in Wellness Kit with Super Negative over colon until symptoms stop. If constipation occurs, use Positive Super on colon for 10-20 minutes. This will stimulate elimination. Follow with Daytime (♥PD WARNING), Nightime, drink 4 glasses of BNW with BAO in 2 glasses. Eliminate all red meat, carbohydrates and sugar for 4 weeks, while increasing vegetables and fermented foods, such as sauerkraut. Supplement professional grade probiotic daily (health food store) for 3-4 weeks along with 2-3 grams daily Liposomal vitamin C. See Nutrition. Term: 1-4 weeks.

Concentration: See Anxiety, above.

Congestion: See Bronchitis, Colds, above.

Conjunctivitis: Eyes. See Allergies, under Eyes, below.

Constipation: Pos Super immediately on colon for 10-20 minutes along with 3 grams ascorbic vitamin C and a glass of BNW with BAO. If chronic, apply ATACC in the *Wellness Kit Pictorial Guide* along with supplementation of additional vitamin C, D and E, and probiotic (health food store). Continue after ATACC with Daytime (♥PD WARNING), Nightime and drink BNW with BAO daily. Reduce red meat, carbohydrates, sugar, and increase fibrous vegetables. See Nutrition. Term: Fairly immediate.

Cough: Negative 2-Stack RBs on left and right lungs. Daytime (♥PD WARNING), Nightime. Drink 4 glasses with BAO in 2 glasses daily. 2-3 grams a day of Vitamin C along with mucolytic supplement such as acetylcysteine or guaifenesin (health food store) to reduce mucus forming congestion. Eliminate milk and milk products. Term: Fairly immediate, but may require health professional.

Cramps (Menstrual): Neg 2-Stack RBs on ovaries and uterus for extended period until pain stops; CVS for same period; Daytime (♥PD WARNING), Nightime, drink BNW with BAO. Term: Until relieved.

Croup: See a physician. Daytime (♥PD WARNING), Nightime, drink BNW with BAO.

Cuts: Wash with 1/4 cup BNW and 50 drops BAO. Neg PW over cut to stop pain and increase healing. Rapid results.

Cystitis: Apply ATACC in the *Wellness Kit Pictorial Guide* while applying Neg Super or 2-Stack RBs over location for minimum 3-4 hours daily, Pos 2-Stack PWs on thymus for 5 minutes several times daily (♥PD WARNING). Follow ATACC with Daytime & CVS, Nightime, drink 4 glasses of BNW with BAO in 2 glasses daily. 2-3 grams liposomal Vitamin C, reduce red meat, carbohydrates, sugar and increase vegetables. See Nutrition, Nutritionist. Term: 3-10 weeks.

Depression: BRT 3 days, Nightime, then CVS all day continuously, Daytime (♥PD WARNING), MET once a day for 5 days (remove CVS during MET). Sleep in completely dark, quiet room. See Nutrition, Nutritionist. Term: Condition adjusts quickly with BRT and then constant CVS placement.

Diabetes (Adult Onset): Often a pancreatic cellular plaque condition with a hypoactive adrenal gland condition. Apply the ATACC in the *Wellness Kit Pictorial Guide* along with 3-month CE chelation therapy. Follow ATACC with Neg 2-Stack RBs over pancreas, Daytime (♥PD WARNING), CVS daily, Nightime, drink 4 glasses BNW with BAO in 2 glasses. Supplement with 2-3 grams liposomal vitamin C daily along with chromium (health food store). Term: 2-3 months.

Abbreviations, p. 178, How to use BioMagnets, p. 123, Illustrations, p. 153, Energized Structured Water, p. 41, BAO Dosage, p. 53, ♥PD WARNING Sign (Pacemaker/Defibrillator WARNING) p. 117, Therapies p.129.

Diarrhea and Dysentery: 2-3 hours daily Neg Super or 2-Stack RBs on right and left colon – apply ATACC in the *Wellness Kit Pictorial Guide*. Supplement 2-3 grams liposomal vitamin C daily, professional Probiotic (health food store) during term and include fermented food such as sauerkraut, etc. Follow ATACC with Daytime (♥PD WARNING), Nightime, drink 4-6 glasses of BNW with BAO. Consult physician if therapy does not relieve condition.

Displacement of Uterus: Caused by birth labor, lifting heavy objects, etc. Negative Super on uterus 24/7 until relief, Daytime (♥PD WARNING), Nightime. Drink BNW. See Nutrition.

Diverticulitis: Neg Super on diverticulum (pain site) minimum of 4 hours a day while applying ATACC in the *Wellness Kit Pictorial Guide*. Follow ATACC with Daytime (♥PD WARNING), MET 45 minutes in morning daily, Nightime, drink 4 glasses BNW with BAO in 2 glasses daily. Reduce red meat, carbohydrates, sugar, and increase fibrous vegetables. Supplement probiotic (health food store) for several weeks and 2-3 grams liposomal vitamin C daily. See Nutrition, see physician. Term: 2-4 weeks.

Dizziness: See Earache, below. Often occurs from high blood pressure (see Blood Pressure), CVS all day. Drink BNW with BAO. Daytime (♥PD WARNING), Nightime; if condition persists, apply MET 45 minutes in the morning, Supplement 3-month CE. See Nutrition, Nutritionist. Term: 1-10 days. If over 10 days, see physician.

Dry Ear: Caused by lack of flow of blood. Apply Neg 2-Stack PW behind back of ear for 2-3 hours daily. CVS 24/7 to vasodilate blood brain barrier until condition clears up. Daytime (♥PD WARNING), Nightime. Drink BNW See Arteriosclerosis, above. Vitamin A and E essential. Term: Until relieved

Dysmenorrhea: Painful menses. Neg Super or 2-Stack RBs on uterus continuously, Daytime (♥PD WARNING), Nightime, drink BNW with BAO. See Nutrition, Nutritionist.

Earache: Check for pus, foreign objects. Use ear pump and flush with BNW with BAO. Apply Neg 2-Stack PW behind back of ear; CVS 24/7 until relief, then daily. Consult physician if condition persists.

Eczema: Inflammation with discharge of eruptions. Wash and spray with 1/4 cup of BNW with 50 drops BAO. Daytime (♥PD WARNING), Nightime, drink BNW with BAO. See Nutrition, Nutritionist.

Eczema, Chronic: apply ATACC in the *Wellness Kit Pictorial Guide*, followed by MET once a day for 2 months along with wash and spray with BNW with BAO. Daytime (♥PD WARNING), Nightime, drink BNW with BAO. See Nutrition. Term: Until condition disappears.

Edema: Swelling and buildup of fluids, generally from trauma. Apply Neg 2-Stack PWs or PW/RB on PPP. Normally relief is very rapid, within hours to several days.

Edema, Acute/Chronic: Apply ATACC in the *Wellness Kit Pictorial Guide.* Follow with Daytime (♥PD WARNING), CVS during day, Nightime, drink 4 glasses BNW with BAO in 2 glasses daily. Apply MET 45 minutes once a day until edema is resolved. Supplement 3 months CE and 6-12 months hGH. Any persistent edema that does not respond to therapy, consult physician IMMEDIATELY.

EMF or Chemical Hypersensitivity: CVS 30 minutes first day increasing 15 minutes each day until 4 hour therapy (15 days) is achieved, then apply ATACC in the *Wellness Kit Pictorial Guide*, then follow with Daytime (♥PD WARNING), CVS, Nightime. Drink BNW with BAO, supplement at 4th week of therapy with hGH 6-12 months. Term: 4-8 months.

Abbreviations, p. 178, How to use BioMagnets, p. 123, Illustrations, p. 153, Energized Structured Water, p. 41, BAO Dosage, p. 53, ♥PD WARNING Sign (Pacemaker/Defibrillator WARNING) p. 117, Therapies p.129.

Emotional Disorders: See Anxiety. BRT for 5 days, then continuous CVS 24/7 (off for bathing) for 2-3 months, Daytime (♥PD WARNING). Reduce red meat, sugar, carbohydrates, and increase green. See Nutrition, and Dental Toxicity, Chapter 11.

Emphysema/COPD: Apply ATACC in the *Wellness Kit Pictorial Guide*. Follow with daily 2-stack RBs on each lung for first 2-3 months and CVS during day, Nightime, drink 4 glasses BNW with BAO in 2 glasses daily. Follow with Daytime (♥PD WARNING), Nightime. Recommended 3-month CE supplementation. New PubMed findings indicate 20-30% greater lung function eating an apple daily for one month. Daily 2-3 grams liposomal vitamin C & 6000-10,000 IU vitamin D daily. See Nutrition. Term: Indefinite.

Epilepsy: Treatment under physician's care. Neg CVS 24/7 for 2-3 months, then optional daytime only. Daytime (♥PD WARNING), MET for 45 minutes daily for 1 month, drink BNW with BAO. Consult physician about progress. See Nutritionist. Important: See Dental Toxicity, Chapter 11.

Eyes: Minor ailments: One Neg PW on temple at end of eye socket minimum 4-6 hours or longer until relief. CVS for term to vasodilate brain blood barrier, drink 4 glasses BNW with BAO in two glasses daily, Daytime (♥PD WARNING), Nightime. Term: several days.

Eyes, Cataract: See Cataracts, above.

Eyes, Glaucoma: See Glaucoma, below.

Eyes, Trachoma: Formation of granules on inner eyelid. Possible spread may ulcerate cornea, leading to blindness. One Neg Power Wafer over each eye 10 minutes – morning and night; additionally apply One Neg Power Wafer on temple behind edge of eye socket, minimum 4-6 hours or longer until relief. Wash with BNW with BAO. Drink BNW with BAO in 2 glasses daily. Avoid hot liquids and sunlight. Consult a physician if condition persists.

Fatigue: See Chronic Fatigue Syndrome, above.

Fever: Apply Super Neg for Daytime (♥), CVS, Nightime. Drink lots of BNW with minimum 2 glasses of BAO. See BAO fever dosage. 2-3 grams liposomal vitamin C twice daily and 6000-10,000 IU Vitamin D daily until condition stops. Consult physician if condition persists. See Nutrition.

Fever Blisters: Daytime (♥PD WARNING), Nightime. Neg PW on blisters for 30 minutes, 2-3 times daily. Drink and wash with BNW with BAO. 2-3 grams liposomal vitamin C, D daily. Term: 2-5 days.

Fibroid Tumors: See Cancer, above.

Fibromyalgia: Important to immediately supplement hGH to resolve low hGH in bloodstream to overcome electric shock/cramps/fatigue – continue for 3-6 months. Use the ATACC in the *Wellness Kit Pictorial Guide*, follow with continuous Daytime (♥PD WARNING), CVS minimum all day, Nightime, drink 4-6 glasses BNW with BAO in two glasses daily, supplement with 2-3 grams liposomal vitamin C, see Nutrition, consult Nutritionist. Term: 4-10 weeks.

Fistula: Abnormal tube-like opening between internal organs or between organ and surface of the body. Generally found in anus or in colon (diverticulitis); pus often collects to form a recurrent abscess. See hemorrhoids, gastroenteritis. Neg Super over colon and 2-stack PWs over anus. Daytime (♥PD WARNING), Nightime. Drink BNW with BAO. If constipation occurs, apply Super Pos on colon for 10-15 minutes. Reduce red meat, carbohydrates, sugar, and increase fibrous vegetables. If chronic, see physician. Term: 3-6 weeks.

Abbreviations, p. 178, How to use BioMagnets, p. 123, Illustrations, p. 153, Energized Structured Water, p. 41, BAO Dosage, p. 53, ♥PD WARNING Sign (Pacemaker/Defibrillator WARNING) p. 117, Therapies p.129.

Fracture or Full Bone Break – (also see Fractures, p. 149)

1. Fracture on trunk of body: Apply Neg Super or 2-Stack RBs over fracture including hip and maintain until healed. Term: 3-6 weeks.

2. Full bone break on hip, shoulder or limbs: apply the Circuit Therapy protocol – both the Neg and Pos Supers or 2-stack RB in the PPP (p. 147, 149) as shown on page 113, three inches above and below the break. Keep the Circuit on for 10 days, then remove the Pos application and place the Neg directly over the fracture. Term: normally 3-8 weeks.

3. Crushed and splintered bones: Apply Neg Supers every 3 inches in the PPP. Term: 6-10 weeks.

Note: When applying over cast, apply Super to penetrate through the cast. Use an adhesive bandage to hold magnets in place. Wear until healed. Daytime (♥PD WARNING), Nightime, and drink BNW. Supplement with calcium, magnesium, vitamins C and D.

Fusion: Pain in spine.

1. Circuit Therapy: Neg 2-Stack PWs 1" above fused spine and Pos 2-Stack PWs 1" below fusion. Wear 7-10 days.

2. After 7-10 days, remove Pos 2-Stack PWs and place Neg 2-Stack PWs directly over fusion for 2 weeks. If any pain returns, repeat step one and two for an additional 10-14 days, see Nutrition. Term: 20 days to 6 months.

Gastroenteritis, See Colitis, above, consult Nutritionist.

Glaucoma: High fluid pressure of the eye. Apply Neg PW on temple behind the end of eye socket, 24 hr. daily until relief, CVS 24/7 to vasodilate brain blood barrier for increased circulation. Daytime (♥PD WARNING). Drink 4 glasses BNW with BAO in 2 glasses, 3 month CE chelation recommend. Term: normally within days, but follow up with CE is recommended.

Goiter: Enlargement of thyroid. Apply Neg 2-stack PWs on goiter. Biochemistry needs energy and balance; apply ATACC in the *Wellness Kit Pictorial Guide*. Follow with Daytime (♥PD WARNING), Nightime. Drink BNW with BAO. See Nutritionist. Term: 2-5 months.

Gonorrhea: See physician for antibiotics. Daytime (♥PD WARNING), Nightime. Drinking BNW with BAO is helpful during treatment from physician. Supplement with professional probiotic to replace necessary digestive bacteria lost from antibiotics. 4-5 grams of liposomal vitamin C daily until resolved. See Nutrition.

Gout: See Arthritis, above. Maintain balanced diet, reduce acid producing food: red meat, carbohydrates, sugar, and increase vegetables. See Nutrition, Nutritionist.

Gums: Bleeding, swelling, pyorrhea. Rinse (gargle) with 1/4 cup BNW and 50 drops BAO. Neg 2-Stack PWs on cheek over gums 3-4 hours daily/all night. Floss after meals. Supplement 2-3 grams of liposomal vitamin C & vitamin D daily, see Nutrition. Term: 1-2 weeks.

Abbreviations, p. 178, How to use BioMagnets, p. 123, Illustrations, p. 153, Energized Structured Water, p. 41, BAO Dosage, p. 53, ♥PD WARNING Sign (Pacemaker/Defibrillator WARNING) p. 117, Therapies p.129.

Headache: Neg Super on crown for 30-60 minutes, BRT for 30 minutes if needed, drink lots of BNW with some BAO – headaches are often from de-hydration. Follow with daily CVS & Daytime (♥PD WARNING), Nightime. If headache is persistent, continue with BRT; lavender aroma helpful. Term: Usually fairly quick.

Heart Condition: If DEGENERATIVE HEART FAILURE, DO NOT APPLY ANY THERAPY – drink BNW with BAO. If no degenerative heart failure: Daytime (♥PD WARNING), CVS, Nightime, drink BNW with extra BAO. CE chelation is recommended; reduce red meat, carbohydrates, sugar, and increase vegetables, see Nutrition, Nutritionist.

Hemorrhoids: Neg 2-Stack PWs on hemorrhoids when sitting, place PWs on underwear one inside and one outside, Daytime (♥PD WARNING), Nightime, drink 4 glasses BNW with BAO in 2 glasses, wash with 1/4 cup BNW and 50 drops BAO. See Nutrition, reduce red meat, carbohydrates, sugar, and increase fibrous vegetables. Vitamin A, C, D and E. Term: 2-3 days. If chronic, see physician.

Hernia: Neg 2-Stack RBs on location for minimum 4-6 hours daily, all day preferred. Wear girdle-type bandage to hold hernia in place during therapy. Daytime (♥PD WARNING), Nightime. Drink BAO. Diet: gentle, soft foods, reduce red meat, carbohydrates, sugar, and increase fibrous vegetables. Vitamins A, C, D and E, see Nutrition. Contact physician if condition is severe or no improvement. Avoid strenuous activity or lifting heavy objects. Term: 3-6 weeks.

Hernia, Hiatal: Neg 2-Stack RBs daily just below indentation of sternum (Daytime placement – ♥PD WARNING), Nightime, drink BNW. Eat small amounts of non-spicy food, reduce red meat, carbohydrates, sugar, and increase fibrous vegetables. See Nutrition, Nutritionist. Term: 2-3 weeks.

Herpes, General: Daytime (♥PD WARNING), Nightime. Drink and wash area with BNW with BAO. Neg 2-Stack PWs on location 2-3 hours daily, 2-3 grams liposomal vitamin C daily + D. See Nutrition. Chronic, contact physician for antibiotics. Term: 10 days.

Hydrocele: Accumulation of fluids around a testicle in scrotum. When sitting, apply Neg 2-Stack RBs on scrotum continuously until relief. When moving, apply Neg 2-Stack PWs inside and outside of underwear to hold in place. Daytime (♥PD WARNING), Nightime, drink BNW with BAO. Term: Until relief.

Hypertension: See Arteriosclerosis. Recommended ATACC in the *Wellness Kit Pictorial Guide*, then follow with Daytime (♥PD WARNING), Nightime, MET for 45 minutes 3 times a week. Recommended CE chelation for 3 months, drink BNW with BAO in 2 glasses. Reduce red meat, carbohydrates, sugar, and increase vegetables, see Nutrition, consult Nutritionist. Taurine and l-arginine to soften arteries. Term: 2-3 months.

Hyper- or Hypothyroidism: Recommended ATACC in the *Wellness Kit Pictorial Guide* with continued CVS all day for 60 days. Follow ATACC with Daytime (♥PD WARNING), Nightime, MET for 45 minutes 3 times a week, drink BNW with some BAO, see Nutrition. Term: 10 days - 2 months.

Abbreviations, p. 178, How to use BioMagnets, p. 123, Illustrations, p. 153, Energized Structured Water, p. 41, BAO Dosage, p. 53, ♥PD WARNING Sign (Pacemaker/Defibrillator WARNING) p. 117, Therapies p.129.

Indigestion: Often occurs from diet or stress. Immediately drink a glass of BNW, then Pos Super over stomach 15-20 minutes and Daytime (Neg 2-Stack PW on sternum) + acid neutralizer (Tums) if drinking BNW did not eliminate indigestion. Chronic: Daytime (♥PD WARNING), CVS, Nightime, professional probiotic (health food store) for 1 week, reduce red meat, carbohydrates, sugar, and increase vegetables and fermented food, such as sauerkraut. See Nutrition, consult Nutritionist. Term: 3-21 days.

Infections, General – Fever: Neg 2-Stack RBs on Daytime sternum placement, drink BNW with BAO and 3 grams liposomal vitamin C + NSAID (non steroid anti-inflammatory drug) such as acetaminophen or ibuprofen.

Infectious site: Neg 2-Stack PW on area continuously until condition stops. Daytime (♥PD WARNING), Nightime. Drink BNW with BAO. Wash any topical infection with 1/4 cup BNW and 50 drops BAO, 2-3 grams liposomal vitamin C daily. Consult physician. Term: Until relief.

Infections, Fungal: Fungal, external, athlete's foot, skin: Wash with 1/4 cup BNW and 50 drops of BAO 3 times a day. Daytime (♥PD WARNING), Nightime, drink BNW with BAO, 2-3 grams liposomal vitamin C daily. See Nutrition. Term: 3-14 days.

Infections, Lung: OGE 24/3, then follow with Neg 2-Stack RBs or Supers on both lungs continuously until condition stops. Daytime (♥PD WARNING), Nightime, drink BNW with fever dosage of BAO, MET daily for 45 minutes. 2-3 grams liposomal vitamin C (daily) and D, see Nutrition, Nutritionist. Term: 3-14 days. See physician if condition persists.

Infection, Urinary and Bladder: Apply Neg Super on bladder for 3-6 hours minimum. Repeat if necessary. If constipation occurs, place

Pos Super on colon for 10-15 minutes. Daytime (♥PD WARNING), Nightime, drink BNW with high dose BAO, 2-3 grams liposomal vitamin C (daily), see Nutrition. Term: 3-5 days. See physician if condition persists.

Influenza: Neg 2-Stack RBs Daytime (♥PD WARNING), Nightime, drink 6-8 glasses of BNW with fever dosage BAO in 2 glasses, 2-3 grams liposomal vitamin C, see Nutrition. Term: 2 weeks.

Insomnia: Nightime therapy very important, CVS during day. Daytime (♥PD WARNING), drink BNW with some BAO. No caffeine or sugary foods late in day, sleep in dark, quiet room, magnesium, calcium and B-vitamins.

Jaundice: Liver problem resulting in yellow coloring of eyes, skin, nails and urine. See Liver, below.

Kidney Problems: Apply ATACC in the *Wellness Kit Pictorial Guide.* If condition continues, follow with 2-Stack PW/RB over each kidney 24/7 for 2-3 weeks, MET once a day for 45 minutes 2-3 weeks, Daytime (♥PD WARNING), Nightime, drink 4-6 glasses of BNW with BAO in 2 glasses to flush out possible stones. See Nutrition, Nutritionist. Term: 1-6 weeks.

Knee Pain: Negative 2-Stack RBs on knee until pain is alleviated, see PPP, p.138. If comfort is achieved within 3.5 days, continue for 10 days; if no comfort, apply Knee Circuit Therapy in Knee Kit or *Wellness Kit Pictorial Guide,* adjunct Daytime (♥PD WARNING), Nightime, see Arthritis, above, see Nutrition. Term: 2-3 weeks.

Abbreviations, p. 178, How to use BioMagnets, p. 123, Illustrations, p. 153, Energized Structured Water, p. 41, BAO Dosage, p. 53, ♥PD WARNING Sign (Pacemaker/Defibrillator WARNING) p. 117, Therapies p.129.

Laryngitis: Neg 2-Stack PWs on throat continuously, gargle with 1/4 cup BNW with 50 drops BAO, Daytime (♥PD WARNING), CVS, Nightime. Drink BNW with normal BAO dosage, 2-3 grams liposomal vitamin C daily and D, see Nutrition. Term: 1-3 days.

Learning Disorders: CVS 24/7, Daytime (♥PD WARNING), Nightime. Drink BNW. Reduce sugar (including fruit drinks and sodas), red meat, carbohydrates, and increase vegetables. Optional Neg 2-Stack PWs on each temple 30-60 minutes a day, MET once a day for 45 minutes, see Nutrition. Term: 3 months.

Leucorrhoea: Excessive white vaginal discharge. Apply Neg Super over ovaries, uterus, and vagina 4-6 hours daily minimum. Apply Pos Super on colon for 10-15 minutes if constipation occurs. Douche 3 times a day with 1/4 cup BNW and 50 drops BAO. Daytime (♥PD WARNING), Nightime, drink 4 glasses BNW with BAO in 2 glasses. 2-3 grams liposomal vitamin C daily and D, see Nutrition, Nutritionist. Term: 3-5 days. Consult physician if condition persists.

Leucoderma: Pigmentation disorder of white patches appearing. Apply ATACC in the *Wellness Kit Pictorial Guide*, follow with 2-Stack RBs Neg on right lobe liver all day for 60 days, Daytime (♥PD WARNING), Nightime, MET for 45 minutes 3 times a week for 1 month, drink BNW with BAO, see Nutritionist. Term: 2-10 weeks.

Leukemia: See Cancer, above. Apply OGE 24/5, then Daytime Neg Super or 2-Stack RBs (♥PD WARNING), Nightime, drink BNW with BAO. 5-6 gram liposomal vitamin C, reduce red meat, sugar, carbohydrates, and increase vegetables for alkaline diet. See Nutrition, Nutritionist. Consult with physician for blood count. Term: approximately 6 weeks.

Liver Toxicity or Enlargement: Apply ATACC in the *Wellness Kit Pictorial Guide*. Then follow with 2 Neg Supers or 2-Stack RBs over (♥PD WARNING) both right and left liver lobes for 2-3 hours daily for 2 weeks, Nightime, MET for 45 minutes 3 times a week for 1month, drink 4 glasses BNW with BAO in 2 glasses daily, then Daytime continuously (♥PD WARNING), 2-3 grams liposomal vitamin C daily and D, see Nutrition, Nutritionist. Term: 2 weeks.

Loss of memory: BRT 3 times a day, plus Daytime (♥PD WARNING) for 10 days, then CVS 24/7 for 2 months, Daytime, Nightime, MET for 45 minutes 3 times a week, drink BNW with BAO, 3 months CE chelation recommended along with 2-3 grams liposomal vitamin C daily and D. see Nutrition. Term: 2-3 months.

Lumbago: Pain in lumbar area of back. See Backache, above.

Lupus Erythematosus: Apply ATACC in the *Wellness Kit Pictorial Guide*. Follow with Daytime (♥PD WARNING), Nightime, MET for 45 minutes 3 times a week for 1 month, drink BNW with BAO in 2 glasses daily, 2-3 grams liposomal vitamin C daily and D. See Nutrition, Nutritionist. Term: 8-10 weeks.

Lymph Nodes: Neg Super and/or 2-Stack RBs on lymph glands and spleen, see Illustrations, p. 153, Daytime (♥PD WARNING), CVS, Nightime, MET for 45 minutes daily for 10 days. Drink lots of BNW with BAO to help detox, 2-3 grams liposomal vitamin C daily and D. See Nutrition, Nutritionist. Term: 2-6 weeks.

Abbreviations, p. 178, How to use BioMagnets, p. 123, Illustrations, p. 153, Energized Structured Water, p. 41, BAO Dosage, p. 53, ♥PD WARNING Sign (Pacemaker/Defibrillator WARNING) p. 117, Therapies p.129.

Macular Degeneration: Eye degeneration often due to low cir-cula-tion (such as diabetes or plaque buildup). See Arteriosclerosis and Diabetes, above. One Neg PW on each temple behind edge of eye socket for 6 hours or more daily, CVS 24/7 for 1 month, then during day continuously every day, Daytime (♥PD WARNING), 3 month EC chelation recommended, 4 glasses a day BNW with BAO in 2 glasses, see Nutrition, Nutritionist for eye supplementation. Term: 2-3 months.

Menopausal Discomforts: Neg 2-Stack RBs or Super on uterus for 3-4 hours daily. If constipation occurs, place Pos Super on colon for 10-15 minutes. Daytime (♥PD WARNING), CVS, Nightime, hGH helpful, MET once a day for 45 minutes during menstruation, drink BNW with BAO. See Nutrition, Nutritionist. Term: 1 week.

Menorrhagia: Excessive menses. Neg 2-Stack RB or Super on uterus for 3-4 hours daily; if constipation occurs, place Super Positive on colon for 10-15 minutes. Daytime (♥PD WARNING), Nightime, MET once a day for 45 minutes during menstruation, drink BNW with BAO. See Nutrition, supplement with B vitamins, Nutritionist. Term: Normal menstrual period.

Menstrual Irregularity: Neg 2-Stack RBs on uterus for 7-10 days. If constipation occurs, place Super Positive on colon for 10-15 min-utes. Daytime (♥PD WARNING), Nightime, MET 45 minutes daily during menstruation period. Drink BNW with BAO supplement with B vitamins. See Nutrition, Nutritionist. Term: 1-2 months.

Migraine Headache: Apply Neg Super to top of head, single Neg PW on each temple & 2-Stack PW on CVS 24/7 until relief. Drink 4-6 glasses of BNW Negative Water with BAO in 2 glasses to over-come any dehydration. Lavender aroma therapy found excellent. Daytime (♥PD WARNING), Nightime. See Chapters 9, 10, 11 and Nutritionist for possible allergies.

Motion Sickness: Neg Super or 2-Stack RBs on top of head and 2-Stack Neg PW on CVS for several hours after condition stops.

Mumps: Neg 2-Stack PWs over swollen locations 1-3 hours. Daytime (♥PD WARNING), Nightime, wash swollen infected areas with 1/4 cup BNW and 50 drops BAO. Drink BNW with BAO. 2-3 grams liposomal vitamin C and D daily, consult physician. Term: 2-3 weeks average.

Muscle Spasms: Negative 2-Stack PWs over PPP location, MET for 45 minutes daily for 10 days for acute conditions. Daytime (♥PD WARNING), CVS daily for minimum of 1 month, Nightime. Drink BNW with BAO. 2-3 grams liposomal vitamin C, B-complex supplements daily. See Nutrition, Nutritionist. Term: 10 days – 2 months.

Nausea: Negative 2-stack PW/RB over stomach, liver and gall bladder for 30-60 minutes. CVS, drink BNW, follow with Daytime (♥PD WARNING). If condition persists, contact physician. Possible allergy testing.

Nephritis: Inflammation of kidneys. Apply ATACC in the *Wellness Kit Pictorial Guide*; follow with Neg 2-Stack RBs on each kidney for 3 hours minimum daily. Daytime (♥PD WARNING), Nightime, drink BNW with BAO in 2 glasses daily, 2-3 grams liposomal vitamin C (daily), multivitamin. See Nutrition. Term: 10-20 days.

Nerve Regeneration: See Nerve Regeneration, p. 151. Follow with MET to stimulate entire nervous system. Daytime (♥PD WARNING). See Nutrition, Nutritionist. Term: 2-6 weeks.

Abbreviations, p. 178, How to use BioMagnets, p. 123, Illustrations, p. 153, Energized Structured Water, p. 41, BAO Dosage, p. 53, ♥PD WARNING Sign (Pacemaker/Defibrillator WARNING) p. 117, Therapies p.129.

Nervousness: See Anxiety, above.

Neuritis: Inflammation of a nerve. Neg 2-Stack PWs over PPP location 24/5; follow with MET. Daytime (♥PD WARNING), CVS, Nightime, drink BNW with BAO. See Nerve Regeneration, p. 151. Nutritionist important. Term: Until condition stops.

Obesity: Apply ATACC in the *Wellness Kit Pictorial Guide*, follow with Pos 2-Stack RBs on left and right colon 10 minutes after eating, daily for 2 weeks. CVS 24/7 for thyroid therapy. Daytime (♥PD WARNING), Nightime; drink BNW. Professional probiotic (health food store or on-line) a must. See Nutrition. Cut down on carbohydrates, sugar, and increase vegetables. Taurine and hGH supplements helpful. Term: 4-8 months.

Orchitis: Inflammation of the testes. See Hydrocele, above.

Osteoporosis: Apply ATACC in the *Wellness Kit Pictorial Guide*, follow Daytime (♥PD WARNING), CVS, Nightime, MET 45 minutes 3 times a week, drink BNW with BAO. See Nutrition, Nutritionist for supplementation required.

Ovarian Cysts: Neg Super or 2-Stack RBs on ovaries 24/7 for 2-4 weeks. At same time: OGE, then Daytime (♥PD WARNING), CVS, Nightime, MET 45 minutes 3 times a week, drink BNW with BAO. See Nutrition, reduce red meat, sugar, milk and milk products, carbohydrates, and increase vegetables; 2-3 grams liposomal vitamin C daily, Nutritionist. Term: 2 weeks – 3 months.

Panic Attacks: See Anxiety, above.

Pancreas: See Diabetes, above. Neg Super or 2-Stack RBs on pancreas 24/7 for 2 weeks, Daytime (♥PD WARNING), Nightime, MET 45 minutes daily. Optional preferred therapy: Apply ATACC in the *Wellness Kit Pictorial Guide*, then follow with 2-Stack RBs on pancreas 24/7; Daytime, Nightime, MET, drink BNW with BAO in 2 glasses daily. Nutritionist. Term: 7-14 days.

Pain: Normal inflammation from injury, stress, or trauma, apply a Neg 2-Stack PWs or RBs or Super depending upon depth of penetration. On limbs, the Proper Polarity Placement (PPP, p. 138) is required. Adjunct therapies: Daytime (♥PD WARNING), Nightime, drink BNW with BAO if needed. See Nutrition. Term: Until condition stops.

Paralysis, Facial: Neg 2-Stack PWs. Daytime (♥PD WARNING), Nightime, MET 45 minutes daily every other day for 2 weeks, drink 4 glasses BNW with BAO in 2 glasses daily. Avoid cold liquids. Vitamin E, amino acid complex. See Nutrition. Term: Until condition stops. Consult physician.

Paralysis, Body: See *Nerve Regeneration,* p. 151.

1) If condition just occurred, apply Neg 2-Stack PWs for 24/3 days on severed nerve (breach location) to reduce any inflammation.

2) After step 1, apply Nerve Regeneration Circuit Therapy of Neg 2-Stack Power Wafers 1 inch above nerve breach (toward the head) and Pos 2-Stack PWs 1inch below breach.

3) MET 2 times a day for 2 weeks very important; then once a day for 2-3 months. Daytime (♥PD WARNING), Nightime, drink BNW. See Nutrition. Term: 3-6 months.

Pleurisy: Sharp chest pains. Apply Neg Super BioMagnet(s) on chest (♥PD WARNING) over pain immediately, once comfort is achieved, apply preventive ATACC in the *Wellness Kit Pictorial Guide*. Follow with Daytime (♥PD WARNING), CVS, Nightime, drink 4 glasses BNW with BAO in 2 glasses. See Nutrition, Nutritionist. Contact physician immediately if condition persists.

Abbreviations, p. 178, How to use BioMagnets, p. 123, Illustrations, p. 153, Energized Structured Water, p. 41, BAO Dosage, p. 53, ♥PD WARNING Sign (Pacemaker/Defibrillator WARNING) p. 117, Therapies p.129.

Pneumonia: Consult physician for antibiotic. Neg 2-Stack RBs or Super on each lung 24/7 (♥PD WARNING) until resolution is achieved, Nightime, drink BNW with fever dosage BAO. 3 grams daily of liposomal vitamin C, follow with professional probiotic. See Nutrition. Term: 2-3 weeks.

PMS: Premenstrual Syndrome. CVS 24/7, Daytime (♥PD WARNING), Nightime, drink BNW, see Nutrition, Nutritionist, B Complex, multivitamin, vitamin D. Term: 1-5 days.

Polypus: Tumor on nose. Neg single PW on nose minimum 4-6 hours daily and/or all night. Daytime (♥PD WARNING), CVS, Nightime, drink 4 glasses BNW with BAO in 2 glasses. 2-3 grams daily liposomal vitamin C. See Nutrition. Term: 2-3 weeks.

Pregnancy: DO NOT USE BIOMAGNETS on abdomen during pregnancy, Daytime, CVS, Nightime, drink BNW. See Nutrition.

Pregnancy, Postnatal: CVS 24/7 for 2 months, Daytime, 2-Stack PW/RBs down diastasis recti muscles down from chest through groin, to help heal muscles.

Prostate Cancer: See Cancer, above. Sit on Neg Super under testes minimum of 4 hours a day, wear Neg 2-Stack PWs on both sides of underwear facing testes when moving. Daytime (♥PD WARNING), CVS, Nightime, drink 4 glasses BNW with BAO in 2 glasses, 5-6 grams (depending on size) liposomal vitamin C daily. See Nutrition, reduce red meat, carbohydrates, sugar, milk and milk products and increase vegetables. After resolution, supplement with 3-month CE chelation. Term: 6 weeks.

Prostate Enlargement: See prostate cancer, above. Add MET for 45 minutes a day for 2 weeks to above prostate cancer therapy.

Psoriasis: Daytime (♥PD WARNING), CVS, Nightime, drink and wash with BNW with BAO.

Psoriasis, Chronic: apply ATACC in the *Wellness Kit Pictorial Guide*. Follow with Daytime, Nightime, drink 4 glasses BNW with BAO in 2 glasses, Nutrition, Nutritionist. Term: 4-6 weeks.

Rheumatism: General inflammation/degeneration. Apply ATACC in the *Wellness Kit Pictorial Guide*. Follow with Daytime, Nightime, drink 4 glasses BNW with BAO in 2 glasses daily, 2-3 grams liposomal vitamin C, see Nutrition, Nutritionist. Term: 4-6 weeks or until relieved.

Ruptured or Herniated Disk: See p.148. Initially, apply Neg 2-Stack RBs on site to reduce inflammation and pain. If there is comfort within 3 days, maintain the application until full time comfort after removal. If condition persists:

1) Place Negative 2-Stack PWs 2 inches above rupture (toward head) and Positive 2-Stack PWs 2 inches below for 2 weeks, then remove lower Positive 2-Stack and replace Negative 2-Stack directly over disk until pain stops, for 2 more weeks. If pain still persists:

2) As directed on p. 148, apply Positive 2-Stack PWS on spine to increase blood flow to separate discs from pinching nerve, and two Negative 2-Stack RBs 3 inches to the right and left of spine to help heal disc and strengthen muscles to maintain correct position after therapy. Wear all three locations for 10 days, then remove all center 2-Stack PWs and keep the right and left applications for another 2 weeks. Reapply center Pos 2-Stack PWs for another 10 days if pain returns after removing them, then follow with right and left Neg applications for another 2 weeks.

Abbreviations, p. 178, How to use BioMagnets, p. 123, Illustrations, p. 153, Energized Structured Water, p. 41, BAO Dosage, p. 53, ♥PD WARNING Sign (Pacemaker/Defibrillator WARNING) p. 117, Therapies p.129.

Apply Daytime (♥PD WARNING) during therapy to compensate for Positive application on spine, drink BNW with BAO, supplement with CMO (cetyl myristoleate) double daily dosage to help regenerate disconnective tissue. See Nutrition. Term: 1-3 months.

Scar Tissue: Due to lack of oxygen in healing. Daytime (♥PD WARNING). Single Neg PW (PPP not required) 24/7 over scar until gone. Drink & wash with BNW with BAO. See Nutrition. Term: 2-6 months.

Schizophrenia: See Anxiety, above.

Sciatica: Nerve from hips to ankles. See p. 148 and Ruptured Disc, above. Pos 2-Stack PWs on lower spine (L3, L4) with two Neg 2-Stack PW/RBs 3 inches on the left and right of the center Pos 2-Stack PWs for 10 days. Then remove center Pos applications and continue wearing right and left Neg applications for 2 weeks. If the sciatica returns after removing the center Pos 2-Stack, then replace for another 10 days, then repeat removal and neg application for 2 weeks. Maintain Daytime (♥PD WARNING) & Nightime during sciatica therapy. Drink BNW. See Nutrition. Term: 1-2 months.

Seizures: Immediate CVS 24/7 for 2-3 months. Daytime (♥PD WARNING), remove CVS for Nightime, reapply during waking hours; remove for MET 45 minutes daily for 2 weeks, then 3 times a week for 2 weeks. Drink BNW with BAO. See Nutrition, Nutritionist. Work with physician under close scrutiny. May require amalgam removal. See *Dental Toxicity,* Chapter 11.

Shingles: Herpes zoster from chickenpox. Neg 2-Stack RBs for Daytime (♥PD WARNING), Neg 2-Stack PWs for CVS & Nightime. Important to drink BNW with BAO and wash with 1/4th cop of BNW with 50 drops BAO. 3 grams liposomal vitamin C daily. See Nutrition. 1 week supplementation needed of professional probiotic to replace colonic bacteria if antibiotic is prescribed. Consult physician.

Sinusitis: Neg 2-Stack PWs 24/7 or minimally all night on both sides of nose over sinuses to draw fluids out and reduce bacteria. Drink BNW with BAO, 2-3 grams liposomal vitamin C daily. See Nutrition. Term: 3-10 days.

Sleep: See Insomnia, above; Nightime therapy, Chapter 18.

Sore Nipples: Neg 2-Stack PW over nipples. Wash with BNW with BAO. Daytime (♥PD WARNING). See Nutrition.

Sore Throat: Neg 2-Stack PWs throat until resolved. Daytime (♥PD WARNING), CVS, gargle with 1/4 cup BNW with 50 drops, 2-3 grams liposomal vitamin C. Term: hours.

Spondylitis: See Backache, above.

Sprain or Strain: Neg 2-Stack PWs [or 2-Stack RBs if needed for deeper penetration] on PPP of pain site until pain stops.

Stiffness in Neck: Negative 2-Stack Power Wafers on location continuously.

Stress: See Anxiety, above. B vitamins, amino acid complex.

Stones, Gallbladder: (or see Kidney Stones, above), Neg Super or 2-Stack RBs on pain site on gallbladder or kidneys minimum 3-6 hours and/or 24/7 daily until pain stops; Daytime (♥PD WARNING), Nightime. Drink 4-6 glasses BNW with BAO in 2 glasses to help flush stone. See Nutrition, Nutritionist. Term: 10-14 days.

Abbreviations, p. 178, How to use BioMagnets, p. 123, Illustrations, p. 153, Energized Structured Water, p. 41, BAO Dosage, p. 53, ♥PD WARNING Sign (Pacemaker/Defibrillator WARNING) p. 117, Therapies p.129.

Syphilis: Consult physician for antibiotic. See Colds. Follow with Daytime (♥PD WARNING), Nightime, MET 45 minutes once a day for 2 weeks after resolving disease, drink BNW with BAO, supplement with professional probiotic.

Tennis Elbow: Neg 2-Stack PWs on PPP (p. 138) of pain site. If pain persists past 3 days, then apply Elbow CT (see *Wellness Kit Pictorial Guide*) for required time. Term: 2-3 weeks.

Tension: See Anxiety, above. CVS 24/7 for minimum 10 days, Daytime (♥PD WARNING), Nightime, drink BNW with BAO. See Nutrition. Term: Until resolved.

Tinnitus (Ringing in Ears): Unless traumatized reaction, condition may occur from allergies, hypertension, vascular plaque buildup, metal fillings in teeth (see *Dental Toxicity,* Chapter 11). Neg 2-Stack PWs on bone behind ear, minimally 4-6 hours daily; CVS 24/7 or minimally 4-6 hours daily, to vasodilate blood brain barrier; if ringing stops when magnet is applied, it is because of the amalgam fillings in teeth which you should get removed. Daytime (♥PD WARNING), Nightime, supplement CE for 3 months, drink BNW with BAO. See Nutrition, Nutritionist, allergies.

Tonsillitis: CVS until sore throat is gone. Daytime (♥PD WARNING), Nightime. Gargle numerous times daily with 1/4 cup BNW and 50 drops BAO, 2-3 grams liposomal vitamin C daily, see Nutrition. Consult physician if condition persists. If antibiotics are used, supplement afterwards with professional probiotic for 1 week to re-establish colonic bacteria.

Toothache, Abscess and Cavity: Neg 2-Stack PW continuously on cheek over tooth/affected area, gargle in mouth numerous times daily with 1/4 cup BNW and 50 drops BAO, 2-3 grams liposomal vitamin C daily. See dentist if condition persists.

Toxicity: Possible toxic hypersensitivity: CVS 30 minutes first day increasing 15 minutes each day until 4 hour therapy (15 days) is achieved, then apply ATACC in the *Wellness Kit Pictorial Guide*, then follow with Daytime (♥PD WARNING), CVS, Nightime. Drink BNW with BAO, supplement at 4th week of therapy with hGH 6-12 months. Supplement spirulina or green algae for detox, 5 grams liposomal vitamin C first two days to neutralize toxicity, then 2-3 grams daily.See Nutritionist. Term: 2-3 weeks.

Trauma: Injury from falls, accidents, etc. Neg 2-Stack PWs or RBs for greater penetration value on PPP (p. 138) on pain site location, maintain for 2-3 days after pain stops to help ensure healing. Daytime (♥PD WARNING), Nightime, drink BNW with BAO for wellness and maintenance.

Triglycerides: See Arteriosclerosis, above.

Tuberculosis: Apply ATACC in the *Wellness Kit Pictorial Guide*, then follow with Daytime (♥PD WARNING), CVS, Nightime. Drink BNW with BAO, supplement 5 grams liposomal vitamin C daily for 6 weeks. See Nutrition. Consult physician.

Tumor: See Cancer, above.

Ulcer: Neg 2-Stack RBs over stomach continuously and apply ATACC in the *Wellness Kit Pictorial Guide*, then follow with Daytime (♥PD WARNING), CVS, Nightime. Drink BNW, bland diet. See Nutritionist. Consult physician.

Abbreviations, p. 178, How to use BioMagnets, p. 123, Illustrations, p. 153, Energized Structured Water, p. 41, BAO Dosage, p. 53, ♥PD WARNING Sign (Pacemaker/Defibrillator WARNING) p. 117, Therapies p.129.

Urinary Problems: Apply OGE, follow with 2-Stack PW/RB over bladder and kidneys for minimum of 2-3 hours daily, MET once a day, for 2 weeks, Daytime (♥PD WARNING), Nightime, drink BNW with BAO. 5 grams liposomal vitamin C first three days to reduce inflammation, then 2-3 grams daily. See Nutritionist. Term: 2-15 days.

Urticaria: Allergic disease showing elevated red patches that show on skin from time to time. May be itchy and can be aggravated by clothing. Apply ATACC in the *Wellness Kit Pictorial Guide*, then follow with Daytime (♥PD WARNING), CVS, Nightime, drink BNW with BAO, 2-3 gram liposomal vitamin C daily. See Nutritionist.

Vaginal Infections: Neg Super or 2-Stack RBs over vagina 24/6. Douche daily with 1/4 cup of BNW with 50 drops for one week. Daytime (♥PD WARNING), Nightime Therapy, drink BNW with BAO, 2-3 grams liposomal vitamin C daily. See Nutrition, Nutritionist. If condition persists consult physician.

Vitality: Apply ATACC in the *Wellness Kit Pictorial Guide*, then follow with Daytime (♥PD WARNING), CVS, Nightime, drink 4-6 glasses BNW with BAO in 2 glasses, 2-3 grams liposomal vitamin C daily, optional hGH for 6-12 months. See Nutrition, Nutritionist.

Weight Problem: See Obesity, above.

Weak Muscles: Apply ATACC in the Pictorial Guide, then follow with Daytime (♥PD WARNING), CVS, Nightime, drink 4-6 glasses BNW with BAO in 2 glasses, 2-3 grams liposomal vitamin C daily, optional hGH for 6-12 months, start exercising and continue. See Nutrition, Nutritionist.

Whiplash: Apply whiplash therapy as shown in the *Wellness Kit Pictorial Guide.*

Withdrawal Symptoms: See Addictive States, above, and supplement with 5-6 grams of liposomal vitamin C daily for 10 days, then 2-3 grams a day maintenance.

Abbreviations, p. 178, How to use BioMagnets, p. 123, Illustrations, p. 153, Energized Structured Water, p. 41, BAO Dosage, p. 53, ♥PD WARNING Sign (Pacemaker/Defibrillator WARNING) p. 117, Therapies p.129.

APPENDIX A

Peak Energy Performance, Inc.

Peak Energy Performance (PEP) was formed in 1996 by Thomas E. Levy, MD, JDM, FACC. PEP took over the blood biocompatibility testing initiated by Dr. Hal Huggins to help determine the best replacement materials when mercury amalgams or other dental materials are removed.

The general mission of PEP is to help those people who are seeking to avoid as much toxicity as possible and reach better states of health. Further, PEP wants to increase the awareness of the effects of dental toxicity on the health of many people, since the mouth appears to be the source of greatest toxicity for most people. Through education on a number of special programs, PEP attempts to help the motivated individual through what can be a very confusing maze of conflicting information, to reach a state of minimal toxicity and optimal health.

The blood biocompatibility test is a sophisticated blood test to help determine on an individual basis the least toxic replacement dental material. All foreign substances introduced into the body will provoke the immune system of the patient to some degree. However, some products, such as the mercury amalgam filling, consistently provoke a strong immune response, eventually depleting the strength of the immune system. Most replacement filling materials have a number of chemicals in them that are very capable of continuing the damage initiated by the highly toxic mercury found in most mouths. This testing measures objectively the degree of reactivity between one person's blood serum and the separate components of a commercial dental product. When significant reactivity is seen with any one of the components of a dental product, the entire product is considered to have that amount of reactivity.

The report lists in categories of **Highly Reactive, Moderately Reactive,** and **Least Reactive** nearly 1000 different dental products and materials, including those used in composite fillings, crowns, bridges, cements, dentures, and other dental interventions.

Nearly all reports have some materials in the **Least Reactive** category from which the dentist may choose.

A **Least Reactive** dental product cannot be guaranteed to be a completely safe choice, but experience has consistently shown such a choice to be vastly superior over random choice or the choice of a **Highly Reactive** dental product.

The report is over 30 pages in length and professionally bound, with some introductory explanatory material at the front of the report. For those who obtain this report, a list of dentists can be provided upon request who are believed to be the most aware and best trained dentists to deal with the removal of mercury and other toxins in a specific geographical area. This list is not generally given to those who don't obtain this test, since many people in the past who didn't use the test did not see improvements in their health or even saw declines in their health after the wrong replacement dental materials were used. PEP strongly encourages inquiring individuals to get as educated as possible on the subject of dental toxicity, since blind trust in an uninformed dentist will often worsen their problems.

PEP provides blood serum biocompatibility testing, as originated by Dr. Huggins, to help guide patients to the least toxic replacement fillings and dental materials. PEP also carries a variety of educational materials and Nutritional supplements.

PEP offers Health Assist programs to further guide the individual seeking the removal of dental toxicity. The life-style that one follows after the removal of dental toxicity is very crucial for good long-term health. Detoxification after a total dental revision is typically very BRISK without any additional help and does not need additional encouragement or specific detoxification measures. An individual can schedule a question-and-answer session over the phone, which helps in the choice of the best supplementation, the pursuit of optimal nutrition and the making of other important life-styles decisions. Typically, standard blood, hair and sometimes urine testing is incorporated into a Health Assist program to give the best assurance that the proper direction is being offered.

PEP continues to investigate what supplements best support the immune system. This area is constantly evolving, and what was best at one point in time may not always remain the best choice. Ultimately, the immune system must strengthen and recover if the patient is to show any clinical improvement. PEP offers a limited line of supplements that it feels best fulfills this goal.

PEP supports the full line of BiomagScience BioMagnets. The proper use of these products is important in stimulating the immune system and effecting the recovery of the patient. BioMagnets are also especially useful in the optimal healing of operated dental sites, which can actually become very toxic again if they do not heal correctly.

PEP offers a full line of ozone generators and ozone-related products. The proper use of ozone and its products can be another valuable factor in allowing the recovery of a toxin-weakened immune system.

PEP offers mercury absorbing filtration masks for the amalgam-removing dentist and dental assistant. Mercury vapor cannot be completely avoided, and these masks are an absolute must for the office that removes mercury amalgams.

PEP offers a wide variety of educational videotapes and also some books on the subject of dental toxicity. A number of prominent speakers have been recorded, and this source of information is invaluable and not readily available elsewhere, if at all. Tapes for both health care professionals and the motivated lay person are available.

Hair Analysis Determines Vitamin/Mineral Overload and/or Deficiency

PEP offers a hair analysis to determine whether a vitamin and/or mineral deficiency exists. Hair analysis can be a very useful tool to follow how well the good minerals are being retained and how well the good minerals are being excreted. Remember that the levels measured in any hair analysis represent only what was circulating in the bloodstream while those hairs tested were actively growing. This means that someone can have low levels of a metal in the hair even though the body level of that metal is very high as long as there was not a new large exposure while those exposed hairs were growing. Conversely, the body level can be low and the hair level high if there was a recent high exposure.

All of this means that hair analysis is most useful when several hair analyses over months or years are considered together. Clinical improvement is sometimes noted when toxic levels that were once low temporarily get high, since this means the body is finally detoxifying and releasing the long-stored toxic metals. Sometimes high levels drop to very low levels and then rise to a normal level. This is seen when the patient initially had a very high "non-bioavailable" form of mineral accumulated throughout the body. This mineral first gets mobilized and excreted, and then the body is free to re-accumulate the bioavailable forms of that mineral to normal levels. All of this means that just ONE hair analysis has to be interpreted very carefully, since high or low levels of a mineral or a toxin can be good or bad, depending upon the above perspectives just discussed.

See all of Dr. Levy's important books on dental toxicity, overcoming illness and increasing health with vitamin C, overcoming toxicity and more at:

Peak Energy Performance, Inc. (PEP)
www.peakenergy.com

SOURCES

ADEY, W. R., Tissue Interactions with Non-Ionizing Electromagnetic Fields, Physical Review 61:435-514

ALEXANDER, H.S., Amer. J. Med. Elect., 1962

BANSAL, H.C., Magneto-Therapy B. Jain Publisher Pvt. Ltd: India, 1976

BANSAL, H.L., DR., and BANSAL, R.S., DR., Magnetic Cure for Common Diseases, New Delhi, Bombay, India, 1983, 1990

BAREFOOT, ROBERT R., and REICH, CARL, M.D., The Calcium Factor: The Scientific Secret of Health and Youth, 1992

BARNATHY, M.F., Biological Effects of Magnetic Fields, New York: Plenum Press, Vol.1, 1964; Vol.2, 1969

BASSEN, HOWARD, et al., Reduction of Electric and Magnetic Field Emissions from Electric Blankets, Center for Devices and Radiological Health, FDA, Rockville, MD, BEMS Annual Meeting, June 1991

BASSET, ANDREW, DR., Protocol for Electromagnetic Therapy, Columbia University Orthopaedic Hospital, Presbyterian Medical Center, NYC

BATKEN, STANLEY and TABISAH, EL., Effects of Alternating Magnetic Fields (12 Gauss) of Transplanted Neuroblastoma, Res. Comm. In Chem. Path. and Pharm., 16/2, 351, 1977

BECKER, R.O., and MARINO, A.A., Electromagnetism & Life, Albany, New York: State University of New York Press, 1982

BECKER, R.O., and SELDEN, G., The Body Electric: Electromagnetism & the Foundation of Life, New York: William Morrow & Co, 1985

BECKER, R.O., Cross Currents, Los Angeles: Jeremy P. Tarcher, Inc., 1990

BEGLIANI, L.V.; ROSENWASSER, M.P.; CAVILO, N.; SCHINK, M.M. and BASSET, C.R., Pulsing Electromagnetic Stimulation, Journal of Bone Joint Surgery, 1983, April 64(4):480-5

Biological Effects of Power Frequency Electric and Magnetic Fields, Carnegie Mellon University, Pittsburg, PA, 1989, grant from Department of Energy, Public Policy Section

Biomagnetism Discipline, Opening New Windows on the Workings of the Brain, Heart, and Other Organs, Research News, September, 1989 Int'l Conference on Biomagnetism, New York University, Aug 14-18, 1989

BLACKMAN, C.F.; BENANEM S.G., et al., Effects of ELF (1-12- Hz) and Modulated (50 Hz) RF Fields on the Efflux of Calcium Ions from Brain Tissue in Vitro, Bioelectromagnetics, 6:1-11

BRADFORD, ROBERT W., RODRIQUEZ, RODRIGO, GARCIA, JORGE; and ALLEN, HENRY, The Effect of Magnetic Poles on Accelerated Charge Neutralization of Malignant Tumors in Vivo, Robert W. Bradford Research Institute, 1989

BRIGHTON, CARL T., M.D., Electrically Induced Osteogenesis, symposium sponsored by Dept. of Orthopaedic Surgery, Univ. of Pennsylvania, Phil, PA, 1989

BRODEUR, PAUL, Currents of Death (Power Lines, Computer Terminals and the Attempt to Cover Up Their Threat to Your Health, New York: Simon and Schuster, 1989

BROERINGMEYER, RICHARD, DR., Principals of Magnetic Therapy, Murray Hill, KY: Bio-Energy Health, 1991

BROERINGMEYER, R. and M., Energy Training Manual, Murray Hill, KY: Bio-Energy Health, 1987

Case Histories of Symptom Relief and Longer-Term Rehabilitation, Nikken Providers and Personal Users, Taped Interviews and Follow-up, January 1991, March 1992

CHINBERA, A.; NICOLINI, C and SCHWAN, H.P., Editors, Interaction Between Electromagnetic Fields and Cells, New York: Plenum Press, 1985

CHOKROVERTY, SUAHANSU, Editor; 49 Authors, Magnetic Stimulation in Clinical Neurophysiology, Boston: Butterworths, 1990, ISBN 0-40990150-2, LC 89-804

COHEN, D., EDELSACK, A., and ZIMMERMAN, J., AppL Phys. Letters, 1970

CREASE, ROBERT, Biomagnetism, State University of New York, Stony Brook, Science, Vol.245, September 8, 1989

D' ARSONVAL, A., C.R. Soc. Biol. 1896

DAMADIAN, R., Science, 1971

DAVIS, A.R., and RAWLS, W., Magnetism & Its Effects on the Living System, Kansas City, MO: Acres USA, 1976

DAVIS, A.R., and RAWLS, W., The Magnetic Blueprint of Life, Kansas City, MO: Acres USA, 1979

DAVIS, A.R., and RAWLS, W., The Magnetic Effect, Kansas City, MO: Acres USA, 1975

DAVIS, A.R., The Anatomy of Biomagnetism, Kansas City: Acres USA, 1975

DAVIS, L.D., PAPPAJOHN, K., and PLAVNIEKS, I., "Bibliography of the Biological Effects of Magnetic Fields," Fed. Proc., 1962

DEVINE, J.W., and DEVINE, J.W., Jr., Surgery, 1963

DI MASSA, A., et al., Pulsed Magnetic Fields, Observations, in 353 Patients Suffering from Chronic Pain, Minerva, Anestesial, 55(7-8): 295-9, Naples, Italy, July-Aug 1989

DRILLER, J., CASARELLA, W., ASCH, T., and HILAL, S.K., Med. & Biol. Eng., 1970

EIBSCHUTZ, M., et al., J. Appl. Phys. 1968

EQUEN, M., Magnetic Removal of Foreign Bodies, Springfield, IL: Charles C. Thomas, 1957

ERMAN, MILTON, et al., Low Energy Emission Therapy Treatment for Insomnia, Division of Sleep Disorders, Scripps Clinic and Research Foundation, La Jolla, CA, BEMS Annual Meeting, June, 1991

EVANS, JOHN, Mind, Body and Electromagnetism, 1986

Field Tests of Descaling, New Scientist Magazine, City University of London, June, 1992

FOLEY-NOLAN, DARRAH, M.D., Treatment of Neck Pain, Mater Misericordia Hospital, Dublin Ireland, Dept. of Rheumatology and Rehabilitation

FREEMAN, M.W., ARROT, A., and WATSON, J.H.L., Magnetism in Applied Science, J. Appl Phys. 1960

FREI, E.H., et al. J. Appl. Phys, 1968

GERBER, RICHARD, Vibrational Medicine, Rochester, Vermont: Bear & Co., 1968

GESELOWITZ, D.B., Biophys. J., 1967

GILBERT, W, "De Magnete Magneticisque Corporibus et de Mango Tellure," Physiol. Nova, London, 1960

GOODMAN, REBA, and SHIRLEY-HENDERSON, ANN, Bioelectrochemistry and Bioenergetics, Transcription and Translation in Cells Exposed to Extremely Low Frequency Electromagnetic Fields, 1991

HABERDITZL, W., Nature, 1967

HALLET, MARK, M.D., and COHEN, LEONARD, M.D., A New Method for Stimulation of Nerve and Brain, Journal of American Medical Association, Vol.262:4, July 28, 1989

HEIMLICH, JEAN, What Your Doctor Won't Tell You, Portland, Oregon: Natural Press, January 1, 1990

HILAL, S.K., MICHELSEN, W.J., and DRILLER, J., Appl Phys. 1969

HOLZAPFEL, E.; CREPAN, P.; and PHILIPPE, C., Magnet Therapy, London, England: Thorson's Publishing Group, 1986

HOROWITZ, N., and STAVISH, S., Pioneering Cancer Electrotherapy, Medical Tribune, 1987

ISAKOV, J.F.; GERASKIN, U.I.; and RUDOKOV, S.S., et al., A New Method of Surgical Treatment of Funnel Chest with Help of Permanent Magnets, Chir. Pediatr, 21/5.361, 1980

JENKINS, RICHARD DEAN, The Healing Power of Magnets, Alternative Medicine, February 1992

KATO, MASAMICHI, et al., Effects of 50 Hertz Rotating Magnetic Fields on Melatonin Secretion of RAT, Dept of Physiology, Hokkaido Univ., School of Medicine, Criepi, Japan, BEMS, June, 1991

KENKO, NIPPON; KENKYUKAI (K.K.), SOSHIN; and MIYAZAKI, AKIHIRO, Professor, Magnetic Pad Efficacy Test Results, Kagoshima Univ., 1990-1

KIMBALL, G.C., J. Bact., 1938

KOLIN, A., "Evolution of Electromagnetic Blood Flowmeter," UCLA Forum Med. Sci., 1970

KOLM, HENRY H., and FREEMAN, ARTHUR J., Intense Magnetic Field, Scientific American, April 1965, pp. 66-9

KOTLER, DONALD P., et. al., "Prediction of body cell mass, fat-free mass, and total body water with bioelectrical impedance analysis: effects of race, sex, and disease" Am. J. of Clinical Nutrition 64:3 Sep 1996

LABES, M.M., Nature, 1966

LEDNEY, V.V., Possible Mechanism for the Influence of Weak Magnetic Fields on Biological Systems, Bioeletromagnetics, 12:71-5, 1991

LEFEBYER, M.; WIESENDANGER, M.; CHERLIN, D., BLACKINTON, D.; and MEHTA S., Modulation of Lymphocyte Function in Low Frequency Electric and Magnetic Environments, FASEB journal, Abstract #2433

LIEDTKE, R., Fundamentals of Bioelectrical Impedance, http://rjlsystems.com.

LIGHTWOOD, R. The Remedial Electromagnetic Field, Journal Biomedicine, Vol. 11, England, September, 1989

LIPPOLD, O.C.J. and REDFEARN, J.W.T., Mental Charges Resulting from the Passage of Small Direct Currents Through the Human Brain, British Journal of Psychiatry, 1964, Vol.110, p.76

LONDON, S.J. and TOMAS, D.C., et al., Exposure to Residential Electric and Magnetic Fields and Risk to Childhood Leukemia, American Journal Epidemial, 134:923-37, 1991

LUBORSKY, F.T., DRUMMOND, B.J., and PENTA, A.Q., Amer. J. Roentgen, 1964

LUD, G.V. and DEMECKIY, A.M., Professor, Use of Permanent Magnetic Fields in Reconstructive Surgery of the Main Artery, Head of Dept.

of Surgery, Vitebsk Medical Institute, , Acta Chirurgiae Plasticaes, Vitebsk, USSR, 1990

MAESHIMA, S., "Magnetic Healing Apparatus," July 1922

MAGROU, J. and MANIGUALT, P., C.R. Acad. Sci., 1946

MARET, G. and KIEPENHEUER, J., Bioeffects of Steady Magnetic Fields, Les Houches, France, 1986; 02NLKM; OT 34 B6124

MATANOSKI, 0., et al., Leukemia in Telephone Lineman, Dept. of Epidemiology, Johns Hopkins Univ., Baltimore, MD., Bio-Electromagnetic Society Annual Meeting, June 23-7, 1991

MIGUSHIMA, Y., AKAOAKA, I., and NISHIDA, Y, Effects of Magnetic Field on Inflammation, Experientia 31/12/1411, 1975

McFEE, R., BAULE, G.M., Proc. IEEE60, 1972

MEYERS, P.H., CRONIC, F., and NICE, C.M., Jr., Amer. J. Roenstgen, 1963

MORGAN, M.C.; FLORIG, H.K.; NAIR, I.; HESTER, G.L Controlling Exposure to Transmission Line Electromagnetic Field; A Regulatory Approach That is Compatible with the Available Science, Public Utilities Fortnightly, March 17, 1988:49-58

MYOZAKI, AKIKERO, Magnetic Pad Efficacy Test Results, Kugoshima University School of Medicine, Japan

NAKAEMO, KYOICHI, Magnetic Field Deficiency Syndrome and Magnetic Treatment, Japanese Medical Journal, 2475, Dec. 4, 1976

NAKAMURA, T., et al., J. Appl. Phys,1971

NAKGAWA, KYOICHI, M.D., Magnetic Field Deficiency Syndrome & Magnetic Treatment, Japan Medical Journal #2745, December 4, 1976

NEURATH, P.W., Biological Effects of Magnetic Fields, New York: Plenum Press, 1969

O'CONNOR, M.E., and BENTALL, N.Y, Electromagnetic Congress Proceedings, May: 25-8 Springer-Verlag Berlin, Germany, 1990

OFFICE OF ALTERNATIVE MEDICINE, NATIONAL INSTITUTES OF HEALTH, CONFERENCES AND REPORTS, 1993

PAYNE, BURYL, DR., The Body Magnetic and Getting Started in Magnetic Healing, Boston University and Goddard College, 1989

PAYNE, BURYL, DR., Getting Started in Magnetic Healing, Psychophysics Labs, 214 Matt Ave., Santa Cruz, CA 1988

PHELLA, A.A., et al., On the Sensitivity of Cells and Tissues to Electro-Magnetic Fields, Bioelectrochemistry Laboratory, Dept. of Orthopaedics, Mount Sinai School of Medicine, New York, N.Y. and Dept. of Biophysical and Electronic Engineering, Univ. of Genoa, Italy, BEMS Annual Meeting, June 1991

PHILPOTT, WILLIAM H. and KALITA, DWIGHT K., Brain Allergies: The Psychonutrient Connections, New Canaan, CT: Keats Publiahing, 1980

PHILPOTT, W.P., DR., and TAPLIN, SHARON, Biomagnetic Handbook, Enviro-Tech Products, Chocktaw, OK, 1990

PHILPOTT, WILLIAM P., DR., Critical Review of Holger Hannemann's book, Magnetic Therapy — Balancing Your Body's Energy Flow for Self Healing, New York: Sterling Publishing Co., 1992

PHILPOTT, WILLIAM P., DR., Comparisons of Theoretic Formulations, Diagnostic Techniques and Therapy Techniques Between Richard Broeringmeyer and William P. Philpott, Application of Biomagnetics, 1992

PHILPOTT, WILLIAM P., DR., A Critical Review and Evaluation of Currently Practiced Magnetic Therapy, Philpott Medical Services, Choctaw, OK, April 1991

Pioneering Cancer Electrotherapy, Medical Tribune, 1987

PIRUSIAN, L.A., et al., IZV. Akad. Science SSSR Biol., S4, 1970

PRESMAN, A.S., Electromagnetic Fields and Life, New York: Plenum Press, 1970

REDFEARN, J.W.T. and LIPPOLD, O.C.J., A Preliminary Account of the Clinical Effects of Polarizing the Brain in Certain Psychiatric Disorders, British Journal of Psychiatry, 1964, Vol.110, p.773

ROSEN, A., INOUYE, G.T., and MORSE, A.L., J. Appl. Phys., 1971

SANTIVANI, M.T., The Art of Magnetic Healing, India: B. Jain Publishers Pvt. Ltd., 1986

SAVITZ, D.A. and CALLE, E.E., Leukemia and Occupational Exposure to Electromagnetic Fields: Review of Epidemiological Surveys, J. Occup. Med, 29:47-51, 1987

SEMM, P., Magnetic Sensitivity of Pineal Gland, Nature, 228(1980):206

SHARRARD, W.J.; SUTCLIFFE, M.G.; ROBSON, M.J.; and MACACHERN, A.G., Treatment of Fibrous Non-Union Fractures by Pulsing Electromagnetic Stimulation, Journal of Bone Joint Surgery, Br., 1982, 64(2): 189-93

SYMPOSIUM ON APPLICATION OF MAGNETISM IN BIOENGINEERING, IEEE Trans. Magnetics, MAG-6, 1970

TAREN, J.A., and BABRIELSEN, T.O., Science,1970

TAUBS, GARY, An Electrifying Possibility, Discover, Vol. 86, 22 pp. 23-37, Apr. 1986: TERRY, H.J., The Electromagnetic Measurement of Blood Flow During Arterial Surgery, Biomed Engineering, 1970, 7:466-72

TRAPPER, ARTHUR, et al., Evolving Perspective on the Exposure Risks from Magnetic Fields, Journal of the National Medical Association, September 1990, 82:9.

TROMING, IVAN, Magnets in Your Future, "Magneto-Therapy," Ash Flat, Arkansas: L.H. Publishing Agency, Vol. 5, No. 4, 1991

TYLER, PAUL, EMR and the Brain: A Brief Literature Review, FDA Conference, 1990

Unconventional Cancer Treatments, Office of Technology Assessment, 1989-90

WEID, ZHORY, The Effects of Growth of Hela Cells Due to Strong Exposure to Constant Magnetic Fields, Life Science Lab., Shenzhen University, Shenzhen, China, BEMS Annual Meeting, June, 1991

WEIL, ANDREW, M.D., Natural Health, Natural Medicine, Boston: Houghton Mifflin, 1990

WEN, H.L., and CHEUNG, S.Y.C., Treatment of Drug Addiction by Acupuncture and Electrical Stimulation, Asian Journal of Medicine, 1973, 9:138-41

WILSON, B.W.; STEVEN, R.G.; and ANDERSON, L.E., Editors, Extremely Low Frequency Electromagnetic Fields: The Question of Cancer, Columbus Ohio, Battelle Press, 1990

WINDMILL, IAN M., DR., PH.D. Facial Nerve Stimulation with Magnetic Fields, Division of Communicative Disorders, Univ. of Louisville, Kentucky

WOLLING, GOESTE, DR., Magnets in Your Future, and Curing Cancer With Magnets, Ash Flat, Arkansas: L.H. Publishing Agency, April, 1988

WUNCH-BENDER, E, The Influence of Static Magnetic Fields on Skin Temperature and Blood Flow in Man, Department of Radiology, Univ. of Kiel Medical School, Federal Republic of Germany, 1984

ZABLOTSKY, TED J., M.D., The Application of Permanent Magnets in Musculoskeletal Injuries, Oakland Park, FL: BIOflex Medical Magnets Inc., Oct., 1989

GLOSSARY

Aberrated Growth Behavior Deviating from the normal growth, such as tumors, cancer, etc.

Amino Acids - See Nutrition, Chapter 9.

Atom The smallest part of an element that is capable of entering into a chemical reaction, consisting of the nucleus, which contains protons and neutrons, and surrounding electrons. Two or more atoms make up a molecule.

Bacteria Unicellular organisms that have an outer cell wall and a plasma membrane. Both aerobic (good) and anaerobic (bad) bacteria exist in our bodies. Produces enzymes and/or toxins.
BiPolar Having two poles, i.e., Positive and Negative; also known as multi-polar.

BRT Brain Re-Entrainment Therapy for neurological issues (stroke, Parkinson's, etc.) and optic nerve issues.

CE BiomagScience Circulation Enzymes are an oral chelation that removes vascular plaques; when used with BioMagnets, removes cellular plaque.

Cerebral Vestibular System (CVS) The area located where the back of the skull meets the neck: the brainstem relays signals to the brain from the spinal cord. In biomagnetics the Lower CVS [on the skin at hair line middle of neck] is often used in therapy for headaches and neurological problems.

Chelate In chemistry, to combine with a ring structure much as a claw would grab an object, such as removing plaque; also to ring a protein for proper metabolic induction.

Chelation The act of using a compound to enclose an element such as a mineral or micro-nutrient to take on a charge to pass easily into a cell for metabolizing; or to grasp a toxic substance making it non-active, thus nontoxic.

Chemical Associations Like molecules that cling together. In liquid, forms grape-like clusters.

CVS Cerebral Vestibular System.

EDTA Chelation A specific sodium solution that is dripped into the body by IV to dissolve and remove plaque.

Electrochemical difference Force determining direction of net charge movement; combination of electrical and chemical gradient. These charges are often referred to as a difference in the potential.

Electrolyte Substance in solution that conducts an electric current. The two main elements, sodium and potassium, must always be prevalent in the system in order for there to be correct cellular transfer for normal metabolic function.

Electromagnetism Magnetism arising from electric charge in motion.

Electron An extremely minute charge of Negative electricity revolving around the nucleus of an atom that can be charged Positive. Known as beta particles or rays when emitted from radioactive substances.

Enzymes Protein that accelerates specific chemical reaction but does not undergo net change during the reaction.

Erythrocyte Red blood cell.

Faraday Cage A steel structure to shut out all electrical and electro-magnetic fields and frequencies.

Free Radical Highly reactive unstable atom or group of atoms with at least one unpaired electron. Free Radicals circulate in the blood-stream and will destroy a healthy molecule or cell by ionically bonding and stealing its electron.

Gauss The unit of intensity of a magnetic field. The number of lines of force emitted per square centimeter from magnet.

Homeostasis The stable biochemical balance within the body's internal environment that results from regulatory system actions, the condition known as good health.

Hypercoagulation When the red blood cells (RBCs) clump together in associations instead of remaining individual due to a lack of volt-age known as the Zeta potential

Ion A particle carrying an electric charge.

Ionic Current Strong electrical attraction between two or more oppositely charged ions creating a current.

Kinesiology. Movement derived from a muscular reflex in response to a stimulus such as a toxic reaction.

Liquid Stabilized Oxygen Form of oxygen in a liquid state. Ingredients vary but are non-toxic. See in Chapter 8, *BiomagScience Activated Oxygen*.

Magnet A body that attracts certain materials by virtue of a surrounding field of force produced by the motion of its atomic electrons and the alignment of its atoms.

Magnetic Field A condition in an area established by the presence of a magnet, or given off from an electrical current, and characterized by the existence of magnetic force in every point in the region.

Magnetic Flux The total number of lines of force (energy) passing through a bounded area in a magnetic field, often referred to as gauss at the surface of the pole.

Magnetometer Instrument used to measure and compare the intensity, direction and charge (Positive or Negative) of a field.

MET, Meridian Energizing Therapy Biomagnetic Therapy to re-energize the nerve cells in the main nerve pathways so the neural signal is more fully carried between the brain and tissue sites.

Minerals See Nutrition, Chapter 9.

Molecule Chemical element formed by linking atoms together. In physiology, living molecules join together to make up all the different cells and elements of the body.

Monatomic 1.) An atom that theoretically is not dipolar or only has a Positive or Negative charge. 2.) Occurring as a single atom (monatomic) that has been segregated and de-clustered from a chemical association.

Monopole Using one polar field only for therapy or fluid therapy.

Mutation Any change in the base sequence of DNA that changes genetic information, thereby forming a new and different cell upon division and regeneration i.e., a cancer cell is a mutation.

OGE, Organ Group Energizer A therapy to uniformly elevate all the primary organs at the same time. Used in chronic and acute systemic conditions of illness and disease.

Peptide A subclass of protein having fewer than 50 amino acids in the chain.

Polarity Pertaining to one of the energies of a magnetic field – North (Negative) or South Pole (Positive).

Rouleau Pattern When the red blood cells (RBCs) clump together because they do not have enough charge (zeta potential). In this condition, the RBCs cannot effectively transport nutrition and oxygen to the cells and waste from the cells. See Chapter 20, Natural Blood Thinner.

Static Magnetic Field Generally produced from a stationary, solid state bar magnet or from a single pole non-pulsed electromagnet.

Taurine A class of amino acid presumed to be a neurotransmitter. Referenced in this book as a diet supplement.

Virus A minute organism [parasite] that depends on nutrients inside cells for replication.

Vitamins See Nutrition.

Vortex 1.) In physics and Biomagnetism, it an is an electron spin-charged field emitting from a magnetic force starting at a central point and expanding outward in a 3 dimensional V form. The Positive (Geo South) pole emits a right hand [chirality] spinning vortex from the magnet polar surface; the Negative (Geo North) pole emits a left hand [chirality] spinning vortex from the magnet polar surface.

INDEX

BIOMAGSCIENCE PRODUCTS

BIOMAGNETS, THERAPY KITS & SUPPLEMENTS

BiomagScience Medical BioMagnets are advanced, state of the art, rare earth powered, neodymium magnets in three sizes: Power Wafers, Regulars and Supers. They are designed and specifically powered for the correct width and depth of penetration required by the therapy. Each is color-coded in Universal Green Negative and Red Positive with raised letters on the Red side so that the therapy placement can be felt when applying out of eyesight. See Chapter Seventeen for further BioMagnet Information.

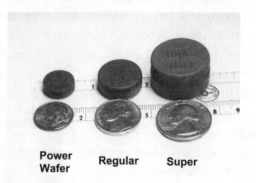

Power
Wafer   Regular   Super

Power Wafer: For general vitality and pain relief; sized about the diameter of a dime, lightweight, powerful and easy to apply. Excellent for most aches, pains, sprains including headaches, toothaches, tendinitis and most localized injuries. Used for simple and advanced therapies and available in the Pain Relief/Vitality Kit, Wellness Kit and Circuit Therapy kits. Single 2020 gauss, 2-stack 2600 gauss. See page 38.

Regular BioMagnet: Used for mid-range width and penetration and Circuit Therapies. Available in the Wellness Kit and other Circuit Therapy kits or separately in pairs. Diameter of a nickel, about 3/8" thick, single Regular 2300 gauss, and a 2-stack 2780 gauss has 18" secondary penetration value. See page 38.

Super BioMagnet: Our most powerful BioMagnet, used for deep wide tissue/organ therapy, a little larger than the diameter of a quarter and about 5/8" thick, it is available in the Wellness Kit or sold separately, each Super has 3150 Gauss and a 22" secondary therapy penetration field. See page 38.

Wellness Kit: Our most popular, comprehensive, and complete Biomagnetic Advanced Therapy Kit. It has twelve of the various size biomagnets required to do all the basic and advanced therapies, self-grip renewable bandage for applications, two water jar magnets for energized water, liquid oxygen,quick reference therapy brochure, Pictorial Guide of Advanced Circuit Therapies, and a copy of *Conquering Pain: The Art of Healing with Biomagnetism* for scientific guidance for over 170 basic and advanced therapies for all aches, pain, soft and hard [including nerve] tissue healing and regeneration, and simple, acute and chronic illness and medical conditions. Used by individuals and practitioners worldwide to help resolve most health conditions, it is one of the most important First-Aid and Wellness tools for every home.

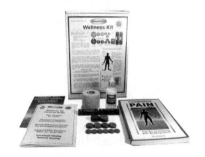

The Wellness Kit contains all the following Therapy Kits:

Pain Relief, Vitality Kit is for relief of aches, pain, and increasing and maintaining vitality. Four Power Wafers and an extensive, informative therapy brochure on how to scientifically apply the magnets for pain and general vitality.

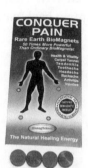

The EMF & Frequent Flyer Fatigue BioMagnet Magnet Protection Kit offers protection from EMF & Frequent Flyer Fatigue and helps to revitalize your body at the cellular level.

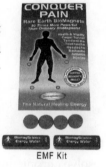

EMF Kit

All the following Circuit Therapy Kits elevate the site's cellular healing energy for immediate pain relief and to help resolve the condition by healing and/or regenerating any damaged or missing tissue including nerve, connective, and all soft and hard tissue. Each kit comes with complete therapy instructions.

Organ Group Energizing Therapy Kit: Elevates the primary organs at the same time (uniformly) for energy & resolution of all hypo-enzyme, hormone and hormone subset outputs to help overcome acute/chronic illness/disease.

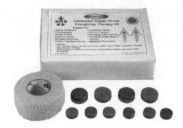

Back Kit: Helping overcome sciatica, chronic back pain, herniated discs, and scoliosis.

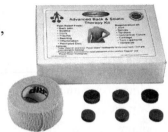

Carpal Tunnel Kit: Pain relief and helping resolve condition.

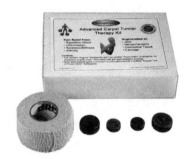

Elbow Kit: Pain relief and helping resolve chronic joint condition.

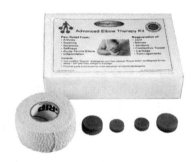

Hip Kit: Pain relief and helping resolve chronic joint condition.

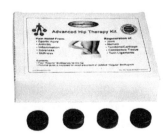

Knee Kit: Pain relief and helping resolve chronic joint condition.

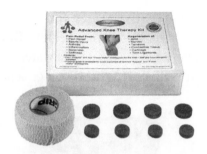

Shoulder Kit: Pain relief of rotator cuff and helping resolve joint condition.

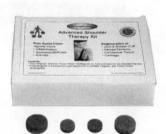

Whiplash Kit: Pain relief and helping resolve condition.

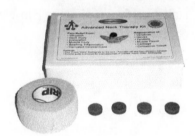

For full benefits, see Products at www.BiomagScience.Net

Bio-Negative Water Jar Magnets: Practical, inexpensive water jar magnets for making healthy Bio-Negatively charged water. Simply attach to the outside of a water jar or sports water container. Available in Wellness Kit, EMF Kit or separately.

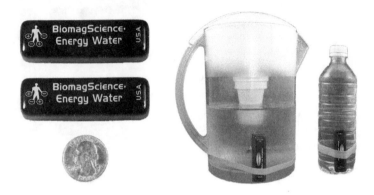

Bio-Negative Water Constant Flow Energizer: Under the sink installation for continuous Bio-Negative energized water whenever the cold water is run.

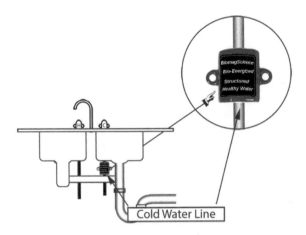

BiomagScience Activated Oxygen (BAO) 2.33 fluid ounces, 1 month daily supply. BAO is one of the safest, most available forms of oxygen in liquid for internal or external use. Oxygen, the most essential ingredient of the body is utilized to cure illness and maintain health and vitality. It is highly useful in overcoming colds, viruses, burns, cuts supplies additional energy and is used in many BiomagScience therapies. Dosage and full information in Chapter 8; comes in Wellness Kit or separately and in an 8 fluid ounce bottle.

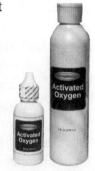

Ultimate Supplement is a bio-identical human growth hormone (hGH) molecule. Used to supplement low hGH in the body, it helps mitosis produce new young cells which help to shed premature aging and become younger. The Ultimate Supplement is also used to as a supplement in such therapies as fibromyalgia and reflex sympathetic dystrophy where the natural levels of hGH are so low, it causes these symptomatic conditions. The Ultimate Supplement is also excellent for losing weight, providing a good night's sleep and all the other known youthful benefits of hGH.

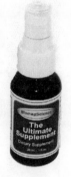

BiomagScience Circulation Enzymes are an excellent oral chelation for reducing vascular plaque for increasing circulation and reducing blood pressure. When used with BiomagScience daily energy supplementation, it reduces pancreatic cellular plaque in helping resolve Adult Onset Type 2 diabetes.

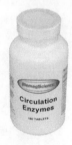

For more information on BiomagScience, its proucts and their additional benefits, go to www.BiomagScience.Net. The site provides full information on Biomagnetism and has numerous white papers and research on why, how and the results of Biomagnetism working on most medical conditions.

The Research section has scientific before and after case studies of microscopy pictures of blood work depicting increased cellular transfer and organ function. Before and after microscopy of free-radical sites shows immediate healing. And case studies of chronically ill individuals bedridden for 15 and 25 years who suddenly start healing are available. The studies literally show individuals' low cellular voltage measurements increasing rapidly within an hour of Biomagscience therapies, something never before seen. If you are interested in further knowledge of Biomagnetism, the website has a lot of important information.

www.BiomagScience.Net
e-mail: Office@BiomagScience.Net